Planning Families
in Nepal

Planning Families in Nepal

GLOBAL AND LOCAL PROJECTS

OF REPRODUCTION

Jan Brunson

RUTGERS UNIVERSITY PRESS

New Brunswick, New Jersey, and London

Library of Congress Cataloging-in-Publication Data

Brunson, Jan, 1977– author.
    Planning families in Nepal : global and local projects of reproduction / Jan Brunson.
        pages cm
    Includes bibliographical references and index.
    ISBN 978-0-8135-7862-0 (hardcover : alk. paper)—ISBN 978-0-8135-7861-3
(pbk. : alk. paper)—ISBN 978-0-8135-7863-7 (e-book (epub))—ISBN (invalid)
978-0-8135-7864-4 (e-book (web pdf))
        1. Family planning—Nepal.   2. Women—Nepal.   I. Title.

HQ766.5.N37B78   2016
    363.9'6095496—dc23

                                                                    2015028618

A British Cataloging-in-Publication record for this book is available from the British
Library.

Visit our website: http://rutgerspress.rutgers.edu

Manufactured in the United States of America

Dedicated to my mother, Sharon Ann, and my aamaa, *Bishnu Devi*

CONTENTS

ACKNOWLEDGMENTS

As I write these acknowledgments, the people of Nepal are coping with a devastating disaster. On April 25, 2015, a magnitude 7.8 earthquake affected a wide region of Nepal, creating destruction as far as China to the north and India to the south. The epicenter was in rural Gorkha District, northwest of the urban capital city of Kathmandu. It triggered numerous strong aftershocks all around the Kathmandu Valley in the days following the earthquake. Survivors slept outside in the rain and cold for several nights out of fear of the aftershocks and collapsing homes. The death toll climbs each day, and several iconic cultural and historic temples and monuments have collapsed. Early reports say that entire villages have been flattened in rural areas near the epicenter, and landslides have decimated others.

As this book goes to press, I worry about the well-being of all the people who so kindly welcomed me into their lives. All of the women, families, and young men whose words and actions I share in this book were affected, but overall the community did not suffer as severe damage as the more rural communities to the northwest and northeast. While many people in Vishnupura are heartbroken over their loss of family members or friends, their houses, and their icons of cultural and religious heritage, I also know well the strength and resilience of these individuals who are no strangers to adversity. While I always intended this book to facilitate their stories being written into the historical record, a documentation of their struggles and successes, I pray that they all have many more days ahead of writing their own histories. Thus it is with a heavy heart but great hope for the future and faith in their resilience that I acknowledge and thank the families of Vishnupura for their hospitality, generosity, and sharing their stories.

As the research for this book unfolded over a span of at least eight years, with several more years of preparation prior to that, there is a multitude of people who deserve acknowledgment. I will try to start from the beginning. For introducing me to fieldwork in South Asia and encouraging my intellectual curiosity in the region, I thank Victoria Baker. For many years of intellectual support and feedback on my contributions to demographic and medical anthropology, I am grateful to David Kertzer, Daniel J. Smith, and Patricia Symonds. For the same with respect to gender and South Asia, I am grateful to Lina Fruzzetti. I owe special thanks to Kathryn March and David Holmberg for their support and expertise during three years of study in their summer Nepali language program at Cornell University, led by the irreplaceable and beloved language guru Shambhu Oja. Equally beloved, and worthy of recognition, is their colleague and counterpart Banu Oja, who directs the Cornell Nepal Study Program (CNSP) in Kirtipur. Banu and the incredible staff at CNSP graciously offered me critical guidance, delicious *daal bhaat*, much laughter, and countless cups of tea. For funding during those early years of research, I thank the Brown University Population Studies and Training Center, Brown University Department of Anthropology, the Fulbright-Hays DDRA, and the Cornell University Foreign Language and Area Studies program. Bowdoin College also supported a critical stage of my research in 2009 and 2010 with the Fletcher Award for faculty research.

I will always be indebted to Ganga Shrestha for entertaining the idea of allowing a foreign researcher into her home, and with time, her family. Ganga's kindness and patience with me over the years is laudable, and though I am a few years older than she is, I have always thought of her affectionately as my *didi* (elder sister). For her friendship, sense of humor, and care over the years, I am grateful to my other sister, Yamuna Shrestha. Thank you for being a caring, generous, and spirited friend. And for their mother, who I now call mother as well, I have such a deep respect and love that I find it difficult to put into words. She understands this, so I will not waste words trying. Without the Shrestha family's support, I could not have conducted this research.

Creating transcripts of recorded interviews is a time-consuming, laborious task that one cannot appreciate until one tries it. For their efforts in assisting with this task over the years, I thank Manoj Shrestha, Geeta Manandhar, and Kavita Dahal. For his assistance in administering a survey to a random sample of homes in Vishunupura, I thank Dambar Pariyar. There are two individuals, however, upon whom the success of this extensive ethnographic research depended. Manoj Shrestha and Meena Manandhar worked as my main research assistants over several years. Manoj was always ready with insights and local expertise, an adept problem-solver, and assisted in numerous capacities. Meena was an expert interviewer, approaching women with an honesty and openness that they respected. Their friendship sustained me.

Several others deserve recognition for their involvement as research slowly turned into text. For significantly shaping this project through their ideas and conversations I thank Benjamin Young and Rachel Sturman.

Bal Krishna Sharma helped me translate several family planning posters relevant to this project, including the one that appears in the Introduction. And I would be remiss not to recognize my colleague Eirik Saethre for welcoming me into the medical anthropology specialization at the University of Hawai'i at Manoa while writing this book, and I thank him and the entire Department of Anthropology for teaching me the meaning of aloha. Christine Yano deserves special recognition for suggesting and supporting a book manuscript workshop for junior faculty while she was Chair of the Department of Anthropology. With the backing of the department, I was able to invite Cecilia Van Hollen to review my manuscript and participate in the workshop along with Chris Yano and Geoff White. The manuscript benefited substantially from this experience, and I am indebted to all of the participants. For her expert and insightful comments on a later draft, I am grateful to Anna Stirr. I also thank Jairus Grove, Charles (Chuck) R. Lawrence, III, and Manfred Steger for their critiques of individual chapters. The thoughtful comments of the anonymous reviewers selected by Rutgers University Press substantively shaped and improved the manuscript, and for that I am grateful. And finally, I greatly appreciate Marlie Wasserman's commitment to this project and her deft guidance through the publishing process as editor. It was truly a pleasure to work with her and her staff at Rutgers University Press. Book projects can continue on forever if allowed to do so, for there are always additional improvements that can be made. Any imperfections that remain in this book are mine alone.

I am the fortunate child of a humble family who taught me to care deeply about others and be curious about the world, but never did they imagine that would lead me to become an anthropologist and conduct research on the other side of the globe. For their unfaltering support of my interests and faith in my pursuits, I will always be grateful to my parents, Joey and Sharon. For supporting me even when I had to take unpaid maternity leave to finish this book, I am indebted to my husband and life partner, Andrew Greene. I also owe him special thanks for his assistance with maps and images. And last, I thank Odin for teaching me the profound lesson of what it means to be a mother.

NOTE ON TRANSLITERATION, TRANSCRIPTION, AND PRONUNCIATION

Throughout this book, the roman alphabet is used for Nepali words that appear in the text. Nepali words that are frequently used are italicized on first instance in the book except for names of people, places, deities, castes, and ethnic groups.

Nepali vowels are represented and pronounced roughly in the following way:

aa	as in *hot*
a	as in *cup*
e	as in *lake*
i	as in *need*
o	as in *rope*
u	as in *mood*
ai	as in *guy*
ou	as in *sew*

Consonants are pronounced approximately the same as their English counterparts, with a few exceptions. The most common ones that are found in this text are:

th, dh	aspirated dental
Th, Dh	aspirated retroflex
t, d	unaspirated dental
T, D	unaspirated retroflex
chh	aspirated *ch*
bh	aspirated *b*
gh	aspirated *g*

In *addition, s* is used for all three of the silibants, as they are not easily distinguished by many of the Nepali speakers with whom I was working.

Knowing which *s* to write in Devanagri script was like a spelling test, according to one Nepali collaborator, rather than recognition of a phoneme. I have not distinguished between the vowel *i* and the long version of it or *u* and the long version of it for the same reason. One justification for taking such liberties is that Nepali is not the mother tongue for many Nepalis but rather a second language, and there are numerous variations on how Nepali is heard and spoken as a result. And last, the extensive conversion of Nepali into Roman script by young Nepalis on the internet and in texting has created fascinating local systems of transcription, and it seems to have affected many young people's ability to spell in Devanagri, despite the fact that Nepali is mostly phonetic.

When using the plural form of a few key Nepali words in the text, I have elected to use the English method of creating a plural noun by adding an *s* at the end. This is due to the fact that for non-Nepali speaking readers, adding the longer plural ending in Nepali (*haru*) might make these key words difficult to recognize easily. In my view, it is more important for readers to learn a few key Nepali words than to conform to the Nepali plural form. In these instances, the Nepali noun appears in italics and the *s* on the end does not. Specialists or Nepali speakers can easily recognize such instances and know that *haru* is implied.

Brackets are used for implied meaning. Parentheses are used for explanation. A pause or interruption in speech is indicated by three dots in a row, while omitted utterances are indicated by three dots with spaces between them.

Planning Families
in Nepal

Introduction

Life in Motion

Scanning my newsfeed for interesting personal and professional announcements one evening, I noticed that USAID Nepal had announced on their Facebook page that September 18, 2014, would be the first annual Family Planning Day in Nepal. Family Planning Association of Nepal and USAID Nepal leaders were photographed carrying a large, blue banner that read, in Nepali, "First Family Planning Day Celebration." Seventeen sponsor logos appeared at the bottom, including governmental organizations, bilateral organizations, multilateral organizations, and international nongovernmental organizations. "Family planning," a phrase that refers to the use of temporary and permanent methods of contraception to space and limit the total number of births, is a sizable industry in the global South. Yet much of that industry is orchestrated in the global North.

Seeing all those logos brought back memories of my first time in Nepal in 2000, when I made appointments for interviews at all the family planning organizations I could find in Kathmandu. It was not a short list. I was conducting exploratory research on women's selection of contraceptive methods. After interviewing the relevant organizations all around the Kathmandu Valley, I conducted thirty-three interviews in clinic settings with married women of various backgrounds in Kirtipur. According to the women interviewed, the side effects of hormonal contraceptives such as injectables (the local version of the synthetic hormone Depo-Provera injection) were significantly impacting their lives. I quickly realized that researching women's contraceptive "choices" was a misnomer; given what the women told me, they did not feel that they had much choice of satisfactory contraceptive methods. Not because the clinics did not offer a selection of various methods, but because all of the methods had significant drawbacks, mostly in the form of side effects such as weight gain, painful and heavy bleeding, dizziness, or breakthrough bleeding throughout the month. Their stories struck me as qualitatively different from the visual representations of target numbers of contraceptive "acceptors" that I saw on family planning offices' walls, hand-painted bar charts and line graphs that were updated as "progress" was made.

Other official visual representations of the work/business of family planning since that time evidence some of the historical evolution of the angle taken by organizations. Like the banner that was carried during the public march marking the First Family Planning Day, posters have been a popular means of presenting information and promulgating attitudes about good health and proper families in Nepal.

On the occasion of International Women's Day in 2002, the Family Planning Association of Nepal (FPAN) published a poster promoting family planning in a major Nepali newspaper. According to the *Nepali Times* (2002), a number of women called the newspaper to complain that the poster was offensive to women. The title of the poster was, "Am I a man's wife or a rooster's hen?" In the illustration, a woman's head is transposed onto a hen's body, and she gazes down at ten hatching eggs that surround her. Emerging from the eggs are the heads of human babies instead of chicks. The designer of the poster was quoted as responding to criticism by saying, "A woman is not a baby-making machine that she has to suffer through the births of dozens of babies just to ensure the continuity of the family line. In my capacity as a man, I was presenting before society the suffering of a mother and seeking a response. I was supporting women, offering sympathy towards the suffering they endure in childbirth." The poster's subtitle read, "A husband plays a major role in ensuring the reproductive health of his wife." Whether one finds the poster offensive or sympathetic toward women, the message was clear: having many children makes one less than human, an animal.

September 26, 2003, marked another "first," the first Reproductive Rights Day in Nepal. A poster designed by the Family Planning Association of Nepal for the occasion framed family planning in the language of human rights rather than population or fertility control. It reads (in Nepali):

Customer Rights Related to Reproductive Health

- Right to know
  Irrespective of their sex, caste, religion, place of residence and marital status, every individual has the right to access means and services of reproductive health and family planning.

- Right to make a selection
  Every customer has the right to freely decide whether and what type of family planning method they want to use.
- Right to be safe
  Every customer has the right to be able to use family planning methods safely and effectively.
- Right to service in a private environment
  Every customer has the right to receive services and counseling related to reproductive health and family planning in a private environment.
- Right to confidentiality
  Every customer has the right to be assured about the confidentiality of their private information in the process of receiving services and counseling.
- Right to receive services in a respectful way
  Every customer should be cared for and served in a respectful and caring way.
- Right to receive service in an unhurried way
  Every customer should realize that they receive services related to reproductive health or family planning in an unhurried way.
- Right to continuity in receiving service
  Every customer has the right to the service they have selected as long as they want.
- Right to voice opinions
  Every customer has the right to voice their opinion related to the service they have received.

This poster frames family making and the continuation of lineages in the language and logic of human rights. These ideals, while admirable, were as distant from women's actual experience as the bar charts of acceptor statistics on office walls.

More than the messages on these banners, charts, and posters, I was interested in women's lived experience and their embodiment of a variety of such discourses on procreation. And as it turned out, many years and interviews later, their "family planning" had as much to do with their sons as it did with family planning messages and contraceptive technologies. I do not mean that what is narrowly defined as son-preference was affecting their fertility behavior, but that sons' future plans of family making were in fact perpetuating marital and residence structures that constrained women's capacity to generate social change. This book, based on almost a decade of research in a community in the Kathmandu Valley, thus offers a glimpse into the complex processes of reproduction and social change in the making.

Anthropological Vertigo

In the early morning haze on the day of Saraswati pujaa, the day that marks the start of spring and on which one worships the Hindu goddess Saraswati, a Nepali friend and I hurried to catch a microbus for the trip to Swayambhunath stupa in Kathmandu to write our names on the walls surrounding the Saraswati shrine. What could be more auspicious for a young anthropologist conducting research in Nepal than adding her name to the countless names of students hoping to be blessed by the Hindu goddess of learning and knowledge? I noticed that more names surrounding the shrine were written using the Roman alphabet (instead of Nepali Devanagari script) compared to what I had informally observed the previous year. If only social change could be so easily quantified and neatly measured by calculating the percentage of names written in Roman script every year for Saraswati pujaa. The ride to Swayambhunath had been an even more cogent example of the difficulty involved in making sense of what is "Nepali."

At the bus stop just down the hill—what would be considered a mountain by those who had not grown up in the land of the Himalaya—we piled into a microbus headed on its regular route around a portion of Ring Road

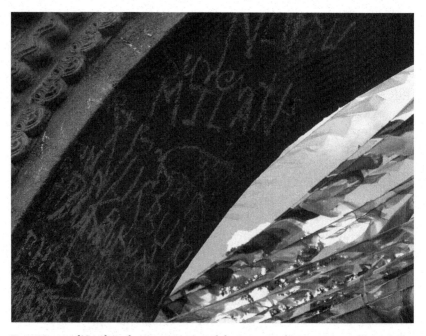

Fig. 1. Names of Nepali students written around the Saraswati shrine at Swayambhunath for the annual occasion of Saraswati pujaa.

and past the Swayambhu gate. Our driver was waiting until the last moment possible to embark from the bus stop in order to maximize the number of passengers squeezed in the back of the tiny van, and thus his profit. The next driver on the route pulled up behind us, honking and thereby insisting any remaining passengers be left for him, and we began careening down the hill. It had not taken much to convince the driver to depart, for the micro already appeared full—and it happened to be full of Tibetan Buddhist monks. There were two major monasteries uphill from where I lived with my Nepali host family, and these young men had either just been visiting or were in residence there. They were fully robed in crimson and saffron dress. I was always impressed by the variety of matching accessories available in those two distinct colors—that day, knitted hats and scarves for the morning chill. As a rule, it is imperative that as many bodies as possible are crammed into vehicles of public transportation, and just when one thinks that number has been reached, two more people climb in. On that day, it was my friend and I who squirmed our way into barely visible slivers of seat among the crimson robes.

As we took off down the hill towards Kathmandu and then west towards Swayambhu, the driver inserted an audiocassette tape into the player. I was anticipating Hindi or Nepali pop music to begin blaring, but since our driver was particularly youthful, anything ranging from Guns 'n' Roses to Bryan Adams would not have been unusual. I underestimated both the hipness of the young man and the apparent increasing speed of global flows, for suddenly Eminem's hit song from the soundtrack *8 Mile* (2002) began blasting. Thus I found myself in a microbus, squeezed between Buddhist monks, on the way to celebrate a Hindu holiday, listening to an Eminem song that was currently popular in the United States. Amused, I looked around to see if any of the monks were singing along.

It is important to note that the only person who experienced a discord between the audio and other sensory information in this scenario was the American anthropologist; the combination of the Eminem song, Tibetan monks, and careening down a hill in Nepal was not particularly notable to the other participants involved. This scenario was distinct from the type of Nepali appropriation of other global media that was familiar to me at that time, such as songs by the Canadian singer Bryan Adams, "Sweet Child O' Mine" by the American rock band Guns 'n' Roses (*Appetite for Destruction*, 1987), or the ubiquitous "Jack and Rose" bandanas featuring an image of the two lead characters from the 1997 film *Titanic* (Cameron). These popular culture products were so commonly encountered in Nepal in the early 2000s, and the timing of their appearance in Nepal so characteristically delayed, that their very popularity seemed Nepali to outsiders. It was the speed at which a song on the hit charts in the United States started showing up in a semi-urban area of Nepal, along with the coincidence that all the passengers were robed monks, that made the microbus scenario in 2005 incongruous to an anthropologist.[1] Yet to the others on the micro, the scene held no irony. This is the kind of complex interrelatedness, a melding of the global and the local, of which anthropologists must make sense in the age of globalization. George Marcus and Michael Fisher noted the early stages of this situation in the 1980s, observing, "Our consciousness has become more global and historical: to invoke another culture is to locate it in a time and space contemporaneous with our own, and thus to see it as a part of our world, rather than a mirror or alternative to ourselves, arising from a totally alien origin" (1986, 134). Now the rate and number of global flows occurring is enough to make an anthropologist's head spin—to induce anthropological vertigo.

As in this opening story, various forms of motion repeatedly appeared during the process of analyzing interview transcripts and fieldnotes. Though this book is a project on the politics of procreation and women's reproductive health in Nepal, motion emerged as a motif as people talked about the broader contexts of their pregnancies, births, contraceptive use, and hopes for the future of their families. I begin with this story of careening around and the ordinariness of the mingling of the global and local as an invitation to move beyond outdated ideas of "culture" or "the local" as static and fixed, and of globalization as homogenizing.

In this book, I take on the contemporary anthropological predicament of studying culture, people, and ideas in flux. This is a study of ideals and behaviors regarding procreation across two generations of women, and several years later, among their sons, in a single semi-urban location in the Kathmandu Valley. The initial period of research was carried out during thirteen months of field research in 2003–2005, and a second stage of field research with young men during three months in the summers of 2009 and 2010. The design of the research unfolded over the years in direct response to the insights provided to me by the participants. As women revealed to me that the practical limitations of the patrilocal family system was the most significant factor shaping their reproductive behavior and driving the need to produce a son, they also wondered aloud whether sons these days would in fact fulfill their obligations to parents and uphold that system. Women were uncertain whether their production of a son would pay off. This was a source of anxiety in a context of declining fertility rates in which women hoped to produce a son in the first or second attempt, and those who did not were left to figure out whether it was worth it to try again. The ideals and future behavior of the sons, then, appeared to have the potential to disrupt a major cultural practice and source of structural gender inequity: patrilocal marriage practices. And while their parents' notions and strategies of family, intimacy, and security may be grounded in more cyclical notions of gender and generations, young people were experiencing such a rapid influx and passing of new trends that they were aware of the transient—and constructed—nature of values.

This book examines the differential effects of globalization on a critical site of social and biological life—reproduction—in a particular time and place. I describe the ways global projects of family planning articulate with local projects of making families and conceptions of the self. In the process, I raise important questions regarding the notion of "planning" when applied to conception and family making and the structural limitations that systems such as patrilocality and economies impose on gender norms.

A Few Key Concepts

In this age of globalization, binaries of traditional and modern, foreign and local, betray their constructed nature and limited applicability to the embodied experience of everyday life. Though it is useful to analyze the origins of global flows of products, funding, program goals, and discourses in order to uncover new and shifting structures and hierarchies of power in the world, for everyday individuals those origins may seem insignificant. In an effort to counteract notions of unilinear, homogenizing flows of globalization moving from economic cores to peripheries, of projecting the theories of the North onto the global South, and reifying the dualism of the global and the local, I fall back on the anthropological method of allowing people to speak for themselves (as much as possible in a text that they did not compose), to contradict themselves, and to disagree with one another. There is no empirical "cultural consensus" (Romney, Weller and Batchelder 1986) to be found in this book, nor experts, nor "authenticity." And though undoubtedly I, as author and anthropologist, am unavoidably influenced by theory from the North, I open up cracks for the people in this book to speak, with the goal of creating conditions for ideas to germinate outside of the North/South binary (Comaroff and Comaroff 2011).

In order to establish a shared starting point for the analyses in this book, there are two concepts that require clarification: globalization and discourse. These are not terms that have a simple, black-and-white dictionary definition. Rather, these concepts are developed through a series of intellectual conversations in social scientific and philosophical scholarship. The meanings of such concepts are open to dispute and revision, thus their definitions are ever-evolving. Often side conversations about a concept develop, or parallel conversations that, unfortunately, do not inform one another (see Ahearn 2001a, 2001b on agency, for example). Thus in order to locate this book within ongoing scholarly conversations and to avoid ambiguous use of jargon, I will briefly outline how others have engaged with these two concepts and how I use them in this book.

Manfred Steger has managed to summarize with precision concepts that have troubled theorists for over a decade. First, he suggests "we adopt the term *globality* to signify a *social condition* characterized by tight global economic, political, cultural, and environmental interconnections and flows that make most of the currently existing borders and boundaries irrelevant" (2009, 8). Beginning with this definition is helpful, for it allows the decoupling of globality and capitalism, its current incarnation. "We could easily imagine different social manifestations of globality: one might be based primarily on values of individualism, competition, and laissez-faire capitalism, while another might draw on more communal and cooperative norms," writes Steger (2009, 8–9). Thus globality is indeterminate in nature; its manifestations are not fixed, nor must it always be associated with capitalism in the future. This serves as a helpful reminder that other globalities might exist, that there are possible alternatives to the hegemonic structures such as neoliberalism, or even biomedicine, that seem to dominate worldviews and analyses of the new millennium.

Globalization, then, would be defined as "a set of social processes that appear to transform our present social condition of weakening nationality into one of globality"; at its core, it is about "shifting forms of human contact" (Steger 2009, 9). What these shifting forms of contact, and their scale, mean to humans (and to those humans studying humans) was what Arjun Appadurai worked to capture by creating his neologisms of "scapes." His term "ethnoscape," for example, refers to a landscape of identity that has a non-localized quality (1991). Appadurai aptly pointed to the increased role of imagination in how globally mobile individuals define themselves and maintain connections to their "cultures" or "homeland." Steger provides a different angle on imagination, and proposes the adoption of the term global imaginary to refer to people's growing consciousness of belonging, in fact, to a global community (2008). How people interpret their place in such a global community and their relationship to it has become an area of great interest in anthropology. Yet how do we study human ideals and practices when so much is in motion, in flux?

Anna Tsing finds method and means to studying globalization in what she defines as zones of friction, areas in which diverse and often-conflicting interactions among various global players produce movement or effect (2004). Others have approached globalization through studying the social life of things (Appadurai 1988), such as pharmaceuticals, as they travel throughout the world and various contexts of meaning and political economies (Biehl 2007; Petryna, Lakoff and Kleinman 2006). No matter what particular approach one develops to studying life in motion, I find reassurance in Sherry Ortner's argument (1995) that as long as anthropologists uphold a commitment to richness and detail they can maintain the "thickness" necessary for anthropological studies in the context of globality.

One way not to study globalization is by repeating the mistakes initially made with modernization theory: characterizing modernity as unilinear, monolithic, and Euro-American-centric (Greenhalgh 1995; Escobar 1994; Ferguson 1997). Rather than assuming that globalization leads to social uniformity and loss of cultural diversity, the underlying assumption should be that globalization is experienced differently depending upon local power structures and subjectivities (Guneratne 2001; Daniel Jordan Smith 2005), and that the so-called local talks back (de Sousa Santos 2008) or is imbricated with the global to the extent that they are difficult to separate (Robertson 1995; Besnier 2011; Browner and Sargent 2011). A lesson learned from anthropological studies of modernization is that such theories are themselves historically situated and therefore require critique as opposed to uncritical adoption and application. Anthropologists' analysis of modernization as projects—rather than some vague force or trend—is instructive for handling today's prevailing theoretical backdrop, globalization (Tsing 2000). This book analyzes global (and local) projects of reproduction through the telling of women's stories in an attempt to attend to the specific social practices, cultural negotiations, institutions, and power relations through which global projects operate (Tsing 2000, 329). Thus this book offers a consideration of the global project of family planning alongside the local projects of planning one's family.

The aspect of globalization most relevant to the women and young men in this study is the way that discourses travel. People, knowledge, technology, and resources are not the only things in motion—so are discourses, or dominant sets of ideas about how life ought to be lived. A discourse is a system of ways of thinking, speaking, and acting, always imbued with power. Some take the form of official discourses, such as the one on family planning espoused by organizations like the United States Agency for International Development (USAID) and International Planned Parenthood Federation. This global discourse is altered slightly to fit various social contexts in the global South, but overall, underlying themes such as lowering fertility as a fundamental aspect of modernization or development are consistent. This discourse gains power at the local level in places like Nepal through its association with the economic supremacy of the global North, complex bilateral relations between nations, notions of modernity, and as demonstrated by Stacy Pigg in Nepal, local understandings of *bikaas* (development) (Pigg 1992). It also gains power through the money that goes hand-in-hand with the themes or messages—aid is provided to supply family planning services, medical devices and equipment, and advertisements promoting smaller families.

Although some discourses may be dominant, all people exist in fields of multiple discourses, and typically many of them conflict. A local discourse on the importance of sons among Hindu groups in Nepal, for example, conflicts with the one described previously of family planning programs promoting a small family (meaning two-child, replacement level fertility), for not every family is so lucky as to have the requisite son within two births. Women thus come to embody, in Thomas Csordas's sense of the word (1990, 1999), these conflicting discourses and processes of social change through the practices of procreating and avoiding pregnancy.

While "discourses" may sound intangible, in fact they are evidenced by observable phenomena. Fertility decline in Nepal, for example, can be traced to the spread of family planning messages, monies, and technologies combined with economic development, urbanization, and increases in the education levels of girls. The introduction of internationally funded family planning organizations to Nepal along with the embrace of development ideals about lowered fertility by Nepali policy-makers beginning in the late 1950s and 1960s eventually culminated in an institutionalized and state-sanctioned discourse about the value of small families. It also resulted in the medical means for limiting and spacing births: the provision of health services and contraceptive technologies. More broadly, contact with products, media, and ideals from all over the world, paired with an increase in exposure to new ideas through an increase in the level of education, has conditioned young Nepalis to expect a world of competing interests and ideas. The extent to which they desire and are able to embrace new ideals given various structural constraints will be explored in terms of a fundamental activity central to family and social life: reproduction.

Previously, scholars such as Appadurai and numerous others working on diasporas and cosmopolitanism had been more concerned with what happens in this respect as people move around the world, but I argue that the world also moves around people. This is evident to an extent in the generational differences that women reported to me, but more poignantly in the experiences of young men preparing for their entry into adulthood. This ethnography offers a brief glimpse of the experience of the world moving around an individual, a phenomenon I call social vertigo. It is the embodied experience of negotiating a state of globality, which is "the context in which many people have to generate a sense of self, come up with the resources that they need to survive, and negotiate social relations with others around them, regrounding into the local context disembedded fragments of social life from both their own immediate life-worlds and life-worlds from faraway locations" (Besnier 2011, 9). Through my follow-up research with sons in 2009–2010, I learned what happens when the local context keeps shifting as new fragments of social life constantly come and go.

History in Motion

The evolving historical backdrop to this eight-year span of field research in Nepal was the Maoist People's War and ongoing political unrest, a radically transformed social milieu from the romanticized peaceful and idyllic portrayal of Nepali life celebrated by outsiders in the past. Rather than writing a historical overview from the vantage point of the present, with all of the hindsight that would bring to the telling of the story, the historical overview that follows is written from the perspective of around 2005. Doing so will hopefully convey a sense of the uncertainty that was being experienced in 2003–2005 within the Kathmandu Valley in regards to the status of the civil war, the violence, and the future of the country. In Chapter four, I pick up the historical narrative again from 2006 until 2010, ending in conjunction with the second phase of research, in order to capture the evolving social milieu of the Valley at that time.

After the unimaginable happened on June 1, 2001—the killing of the royal family, beloved by many—the political situation slowly deteriorated until the point that the international community began worrying and whispering about Nepal becoming a failed state in 2005. The late King Birendra had been one of the more well-liked rulers during his reign from 1972 up until the tragedy in 2001, and some believe his leadership and popularity sustained Nepal through its difficult years as a fledgling democratic constitutional monarchy in the 1990s, reportedly plagued by corrupt politicians and deals. After much political pressure King Birendra granted a multi-party system of governance in 1990, but Nepal technically remained a Hindu kingdom because of the continued role of the monarchy in governance and its control over the country's army. After Gyanendra, the much less popular brother of the late Birendra, took over as king, a triangular stalemate developed between the Maoists, the King, and the political parties.[2] The Maoist People's War had already been in progress for six years at the time of the royal tragedy, but the occasional ceasefire and failed peace talks notwithstanding, it began to intensify and gain momentum from that point through 2007.[3]

During my eleven consecutive months of field research beginning in September 2003, there were frequent interruptions to daily life caused by the People's War and political parties. Protest marches in the streets (*julus*), which sometimes involved huge crowds, created snarls of angry traffic as vehicles took to the backstreets and side alleys in search of a way around the problem. These protests often were peaceful demonstrations with signs and slogans, but sometimes involved throwing stones at security forces and police, carrying burning torches or effigies through the streets, ransacking university administrative offices, and almost always stopping traffic and making passersby nervous. The police met more aggressive demonstrations with tear gas and beatings with batons.[4]

There were also frequent transportation and business strikes (*bandha*), sometimes called by the Maoists and sometimes by the political parties. Outwardly a one-day bandha could seem like a holiday, with entire families spending the day together at home, shops closed, and children playing in the unusually empty, quiet streets. But the absence of noise during the day always created a distinct and palpable eeriness. Anyone operating a vehicle (other than emergency vehicles) did so in spite of the threat that they would be attacked, or located and harassed at a later date by noting down the license plate number. Much more than the one-day bandha, several three-day and even a five-day bandha had dire implications for the Kathmandu Valley. The great majority of produce that supported the approximately one million people living there (in 2003–2004) was brought into the valley by transport truck primarily along one major highway, and a bandha lasting several days threatened food supplies. During those times the Newari family of which I was a part turned to the limited selection of produce in their backyard garden plot since we lived in a more rural area above the valley on the northern rim. Those in the community without gardens and those in urban areas faced price hikes on vegetables and a selection of increasingly ripe/rotten produce. And as in all situations of scarcity, the most impoverished individuals were the people who suffered the most during bandhas, such as those who depended on daily wages from labor in order to purchase that day's meal. The Maoists also occasionally deployed small bombs in various public places such as the main bus station in central Kathmandu, in front of the Parliament building, and in forms of public transportation in order to enforce a sense of fear. This description applies to the Kathmandu Valley; what was happening in the rural areas, and especially the western regions, was difficult to ascertain at the time. News reports from rural areas were scarce and questionable given the lack of a free press. These disturbing political events and disruptions of life became somewhat normalized over time, but not without people regularly expressing their longing for the old days.

When I arrived in Kathmandu for two months of follow-up research on the evening of March 31, 2005, the very next morning King Gyanendra issued a surprise statement on the state-sponsored television channel declaring an indefinite state of emergency that suspended fundamental rights like free speech, free press, and the right to privacy.

The international airport was immediately shut down, and all communication lines were cut, including telephone lines, mobile phones, and all internet connections. Satellite phones were the only way to communicate with the outside world from within Nepal. I had to request the American Embassy to send an email on my behalf to notify my family that I had arrived in Nepal and was alright. The King also sacked the coalition government and dissolved the Parliament, claiming that the political parties had failed Nepal by not resolving the matter of elections or the conflict with the Maoists. This was actually the second time King Gyanendra had dismissed Parliament—a repeat of events from October 2002, down to the detail of dismissing the same prime minister. But this time, because of the state of emergency and revocation of rights, the public understood the potential for danger for common citizens. Human rights abuses abounded on the part of the king's security forces and army as well as by the Maoists, and many people feared being kidnapped or "disappeared." Political figures, activists, journalists, and even professors were arrested and held without being told why or how long they would be kept in captivity. Family members were taken in the middle of the night by plain-clothed men. Reports of torture and rape were common. An Amnesty International press release dated February 10, 2006, stated that, "Ten years of war and political instability have turned the human rights situation in Nepal into one of the worst in the world."

In the community where I lived and worked, these events seemed strangely removed, although there were traces all around. The prime minister's house, for example, was in sight from the rooftop patio of the house where I lived, and security was often tight on the main road leading past his house up the mountainside. The distance that separated the small town, literally at the end of the road, from Kathmandu below also sometimes seemed much greater than it was. One spring night when the electricity had gone out (as it often did), I went up to the rooftop to take down my clothes from the line on the flat rooftop patio (*kousi*) where they had dried earlier in the sun. As I reached the top of the compact iron stairs, I gasped at the expanse of darkness in the valley below. The entire Kathmandu Valley was without power. Usually the lights from Kathmandu twinkled like stars through the haze and smog in the valley below, and blackouts were confined to particular areas. I cannot describe the feeling of nervous anticipation and fear that that darkness engendered. It was if the entire city of Kathmandu and its commanding sprawl were gone. I immediately feared that the Maoists were somehow responsible, but I was wrong. I never did find out what caused such an extensive blackout, but it was something much simpler and more mundane than the possibility that sprung to our minds during such a time of stress.

So rather than the events of the People's War seeming distant, it would be more accurate to say that the fear of something bad happening was tucked conveniently and pragmatically out of sight as people in the Kathmandu Valley continued on with their daily concerns and responsibilities as best they could. Most of the changes brought about by the insurgency and the emergency came in the form of inconveniences and a feeling of foreboding for common people in the community, rather than violence.[5] The armed security forces in their blue camouflage uniforms along the streets of Kathmandu became a familiar sight, as did the routine of checkpoints, strikes, and protests. Cadres of young army men riding in the back of a truck along the streets of the capital city would position themselves facing outwards with guns poised, either ready for an attack or to make an impression. This meant that for people on motorcycles, which outnumbered cars on the road, there were rifles pointed directly at face level as they drove behind the truck or passed it. It is unnerving to have a rifle pointed directly at one's face from only a few feet away as one rides on a motorcycle through busy, unpredictable traffic. On one afternoon a man in street clothes with a bandana covering his face, armed with a rifle, searched our house after claiming he and his partner were police officers on a routine check. These were the types of minor unsettling incidences that I observed firsthand while conducting research in the Valley during troubled times.[6]

Moving Forward

Looking forward, the next chapter, "Intersections: Gender, Class, and Caste in Nepal," introduces the setting of research and some important considerations when conducting research in this area of the world. I walk the reader through the village, past the busy, dusty bus stop and tea stalls of the bazaar, up the mountainside to where houses are spread out and life is decidedly more agricultural than a mere ten minutes down the road. Ethnography involves intersubjective encounters and more than "just facts" (Abu-Lughod 1993), however I use a mixed methods approach because it captures the novel ways that caste, class, and gender interact in this setting. The chapter showcases the significance of intersectionality through telling the stories of a few women's life situations, revealing new evidence that bears on debates about the role of caste, class, and gender hierarchies in contemporary South Asia.

If caste and class have bearing on women's lives, so does their position in the life course. One mother-in-law described the role of women by using the trope of a potter's wheel. With each generation in a household, women circulate out of their natal homes and into the homes of their husbands. Through this metaphor, she emphasized that even seemingly imposing mothers-in-law are not of the household, and women across generations in fact share this characteristic. Chapter two, "Like a Potter's Wheel": From Daughters to Mothers-in-Law, provides insight into the embodied experience of women in different stages of this process, supporting dominant narratives about the experience of young daughters-in-law while disputing those about aging mothers-in-law. The shortcoming of the mother-in-law's trope is the same one present in life cycle analyses—it presents life stages in a timeless way. This observation sets up the next chapter, which provides an analysis that takes into account the specific historical processes that impact women's subjectivities.

Chapter three, The Elusive "Small, Happy Family," is framed by a brief critical analysis of the global discourses—in the academy and the international development community—on women, development, and family planning and their evolution over time. I examine how discourses on family planning impinge upon Nepali women's lives, arguing for an approach to understanding reproductive behavior that allows for the unfolding and improvisational process of reflection and figuring out one's position through speech, action, and inaction. In a scenario in which women are caught between conflicting discourses of smaller families and the importance of producing a son, reproductive behavior can be a process of trying things out—or even stalling—in order to test limits and options. Despite many verbal statements to the contrary, ultimately young, sonless women admitted they were unable to escape the need for a son and the ideal of the multi-generational joint family. Observing their teenage sons' behavior, however, a few women wondered aloud whether sons these days would actually be of any real value.

Five years after the research described in the previous chapters, many of the sons of these women, along with their peers, were poised for major cultural and demographic events such as marriage. These young men had grown up during the Maoist insurgency and come of age in a time of political instability and dramatic social change. This particular history, combined with the more general condition of growing up in an age of globality, led to the experience of what I call social vertigo. In Chapter four, I define social vertigo as a subjectivity in which the high number and short tenure of circulating discourses result in a sense of everything being in motion; the ground spins. For young men of the middle class who had time to reflect on this experience, social vertigo resulted in the ability to see through the constant parade of styles, trends, political and social movements, and the proclaimed newness of things—whether the latest style in jeans or "New Nepal." Trends become evident as such, as passing fads, and discourses become exposed. In this new subjectivity, young men asserted their commitment to a tradition that would appear to be no different from the many others that they easily dismissed—the joint family. Though this revelation would come as a surprise to the women of their mothers' generation, commitment to living with and caring for one's parents was a way of maintaining one's footing. Young men expressed intentions of loyalty in return for their parents raising them, but also the advantages of the emotional, financial, and practical support they would continue to receive from living with their parents. The desire for independence and individualism that increasingly characterizes the political and social milieu in urban Nepal did not extend to these young men's notions of familial relationships.

The ethnography thus captures snapshots over the years of multiple generations and genders dealing with global and local pressures to reproduce in socially prescribed ways. I apply intersectionality as an analytic tool to demonstrate how locally significant power structures combine to impact women's lived experience.[7] However, I argue that intersectionality alone is insufficient in analyzing women's projects of reproduction. Intersectional analysis results in a static portrayal of obstacles and privileges, while the Nepali women I interviewed were engaged in a complex creative process. By this I mean to acknowledge their agency along with structural limitations, but I sidestep debates of agency and resistance and analyze their "projects" on their own terms as they took shape and evolved over time.[8] The book also imparts a sense of the vertigo experienced by the upcoming generation as a result of competing discourses, rapid social change, and influx of trends. Ultimately, young men viewed the family as a place of refuge from the dizzying shifts in values that were occurring around them, and their own ideals regarding their reproductive futures did not appear so different from those of their mothers.

1

Intersections

Gender, Class, and Caste in Nepal

Arriving in Vishnupura from Kathmandu, the bus stops in the social and economic center of the sprawling town.[1] Here the streets are lined with *chiya* (tea) stalls—one-room snack shacks of sorts with fried treats, *momos* (steamed dumplings) and *chaau-chaau* (ramen noodles, Nepali style) that sometimes double as a poor-man's bar—and a variety of open-air shops offering all the services one might possibly need, though on a small scale. A surprisingly diverse array of goods could be produced upon request at even the smallest one-room hardware store or medical shop. The main intersection in the bazaar is flanked on one side by the row of buses and micros waiting to turn around and head back to Kathmandu with their returning passengers (mostly human, but an occasional goat or sack of rice or vegetables was not uncommon). Much of the bazaar has been built up around a famous Hindu temple, and the temple grounds and make-shift stalls selling various religious artifacts necessary for *pujaa* (making an offering in an act of devotion or worship) dominate a large portion of the bazaar. Stalls filled with vivid flowers, fruit, uncooked rice, leaf plates, and multicolored braided string necklaces create a colorful approach to the temple entrances, mostly serving the many out-of-town devotees who need to purchase these items upon arrival.

I lived across the street from the *mandir* (temple) in a four-story concrete building with the standard rooftop patio (*kousi*). The ground floor of the building was rented to a momo stall and a bangle shop, the second floor rooms to renters, and the third and fourth floors were the home of a Nepali family who over a decade became my second or "adopted" family. This spatial arrangement is typical for the buildings in the bazaar, as was the rectangular, concrete building style. It is common to see bundles of iron rods sticking out of the top of a single or two-storied home, a sign that the family could not afford additional levels at that time but has plans for another floor. Home loans were unheard of, so families built and purchased as cash became available. The flat, open patios on the roofs of the building were the location of many daily activities such as drying chilies or wheat, hanging clothes to dry, or doing any activity that could be taken outside for the warmth of the sunshine during the winter months. My adopted Nepali family, like most families in the area, did not bother with the portable heaters that were available on the market at that time, so escaping the penetrating chill of indoors during the day was a great pleasure.

The kousi was also the perfect location for watching the world go by, a most appropriate phrase to describe observing the daily movement of people and goods from a house located on the only road leading down into the bazaar and toward Kathmandu from the upper regions of the Village Development Committee (VDC, an unincorporated rural area composed of nine wards, less developed than a Municipality). From this vantage point, the street and the temple grounds were below. This meant that the music played by hired bands for wedding processions would beckon from the street below, especially during wedding season. All-night sessions—sometimes lasting several days—of special musical praises to the gods (*bhajan*) were clearly audible from the house. This ceaseless singing/chanting, usually by a priest and accompanied by a harmonium, was projected by a loud speaker. I dared wonder aloud once or twice if god, too, did not have to sleep.

While having our morning cups of chiya leaning on the wall of the kousi, we would discuss the parade of uniformed school children of all ages in their pleated skirts, slacks, and ties holding hands or teasing one another, men and women with wage-earning or salaried jobs hurrying to reach the office on time, and a handful of expatriate families in their sport utility vehicles avoiding potholes and pedestrians, as they all made their way down to various destinations in the valley below. Another fixture on the street below in the early days of this research in 2003, though her presence was not as predictable as the flow of students and workers, was a homeless woman who, according to locals, had multiple personalities who spoke different languages. Her rants while standing on the corner became part of the normal life of the street, until one day she was simply gone. Gangs of street dogs prowled the street and alleyways, looking for food and defending their territory against newcomers. During the hot season just prior to the monsoon rains, whiffs of putrid air would circulate around the bazaar from a combination of garbage and human waste. In 2003–2004 there were open gutters lining the street into which sewage sometimes "leaked" or was improperly disposed. (An underground pipe was installed by 2005). The coming and going of tourists on special holidays associated with the mandir, along with community events on the temple grounds on special occasions, were also part of the normal progression of weeks, months, and years. During the harvest season for wheat, one or two enterprising families utilized the vehicular traffic on the paved road in front of their houses to separate the wheat from the chaff. Thus the street was a stage to many social interactions and routines.

The paved road around the mandir gave way to dirt as one traveled farther up the mountainside. However, with the rapid pace of development in this community, a project to pave it had begun by my return in 2005, and by 2010 even the steeper, less populated road that runs roughly parallel to it had been partially paved. As one heads uphill, the houses become more spread out, mud and brick houses of the traditional architectural style become more plentiful, and agricultural fields and boulders begin to dominate the landscape. And yet, of course the community will continue to grow, and these rural attributes are likely to disappear. In 2003–2004, the buying and selling of land was one of the most profitable businesses available to locals. The real estate in the upper region of this area was coveted by wealthy Nepali and expatriate families alike. The land overlooked the Kathmandu Valley, it was above the layer of air pollution that plagued the valley, and the nearby mountain ridge promised a lack of development on one side. In addition, the hot season was several degrees cooler than

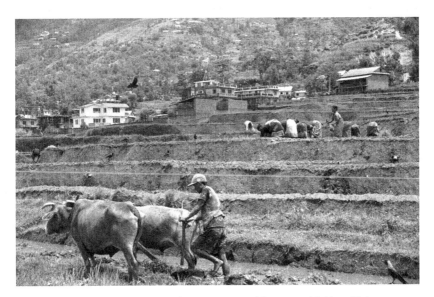

Fig. 2. A man plows and women plant rice in one of the terraced fields in Vishnupura.

in the valley floor below because of a combination of several factors, not excluding the altitude and the partial blockage of the morning and evening sun by the surrounding ridges. The increase in the value of land resulted in some long-established local families selling their land for a substantial windfall of cash and experiencing a dramatic change in lifestyle, and in the irony of some families who continued their agricultural lifestyle living in poverty on land worth more than they would otherwise see in a lifetime.

The two roads that travel up the mountainside lie in the stretch of land that has the least intensity in slope, and several side roads jut off in either direction. After a short stretch of flat land on either side of the roads, the incline gradually becomes sharper. In 2003 only footpaths winded up these steep inclines, and a walk to or from the bazaar would take approximately thirty–forty minutes in one direction. Each year when I return, more roads have been paved and more houses have sprung up. Despite signs of rapid development, as of 2012 these higher, more remote areas (colloquially referred to simply as "*maathi*," or "up there") still retained a more rural feel and way of life than the bazaar below.

As an anthropologist, I was drawn to this location for its geographic and demographic characteristics. Geographically this VDC is located at the periphery of the Kathmandu Valley, poised on the rim of the valley with the urban metropolis below and the rural expanse beyond the ridge of mountains that encase the valley. Its in-between status, neither a village

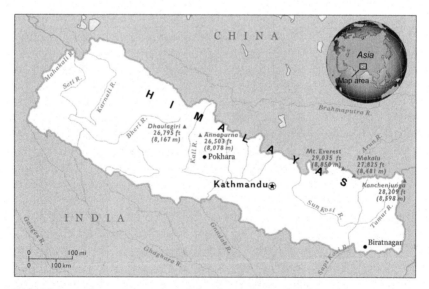

Fig. 3. The research community sits just below the northern ridge of the Kathmandu Valley in Nepal.

nor a city, meant that it was a middle ground between two extremes that dominate life in Nepal—that of crowded, cosmopolitan Kathmandu (and a few other such cities) and rural, remote, "village" Nepal. Vishnupura's location and semi-urban status made it an ideal place to study social change. It was a manageable microcosm of social change in motion.

The other reason for selecting this site was the distribution of ethnic and caste groups represented in its population. For its small size, Nepal contains an impressive amount of ethnic and linguistic diversity. Limiting the present study to a cultural subgroup of the nation's diverse population was necessary in order to limit cultural variation. I chose the group whose ideologies had been dominant both politically and socially since the consolidation of the country in 1768 until the overthrow of the Hindu monarchy in 2007: *Parbatiya* (hill dwelling, referring to the middle hills region of Nepal) Hindus. This group includes Brahmin (or Bahun), Chhetri, Thakuri, and Dalit.[2] The Parbatiya group is distinct because of its social and linguistic history, but ultimately it is a loose approximation of a cultural group that is heterogeneous because of the *jaats* or subgroups (often glossed as "castes") that comprise it as well as the increasingly porous boundaries that demarcate it. In order to avoid the reification of the name "Parbatiya" as a "culture," I prefer to use the more accessible and general term, "Hindu-caste."

After obtaining census records from the Central Bureau of Statistics and charting the ethnic breakdown of a few potential research sites, Vishnupura emerged as an ideal site because of its large percentage of Hindu-caste residents (unlike many of the predominantly Newar towns around the edges of the Kathmandu Valley).[3] It also turned out that this location was not directly affected by recruiting or violence associated with the ongoing Maoist People's War, which was a significant barrier to doing research outside of the Kathmandu Valley at the time.

During the thirteen months of research carried out between 2003 and 2005, I used a combination of qualitative and quantitative methods that incorporated ongoing participant observation, the enumeration of households and a survey of a random sample of households, the selection of thirty case studies representing a range of important cultural and economic factors, interviews and observations at the local sub-health post and the two hospitals used by locals, and immersion in family and community life by becoming the paying guest of a local Newari family and participating in daily life and rituals. My status as a fictive daughter of a local family provided me with credibility in the community and significantly aided in my acceptance. And, more importantly for the long term, I gained what has truly become a second family over many years of visiting and sharing life's joys and setbacks.

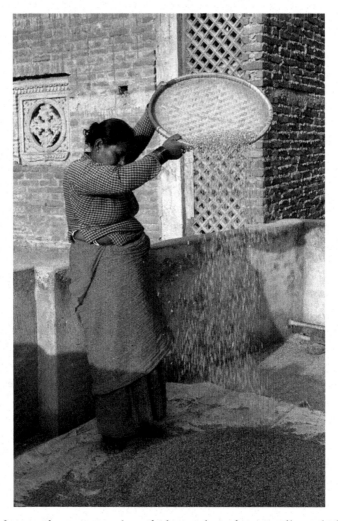

Fig. 4. My fictive mother uses a *naanglo* to sift wheat on the rooftop patio of her multiple story home.

In the initial months of the project, I mapped and enumerated house-holds (N = 794) of the two most populous political sections (wards) of the village, and surveyed a random sample of 248 households for basic demographic, household history, and birth information. The number 250 was selected as a number that would result in statistically significant descriptive statistics for the population of households in the two wards.[4] The data gathered in the survey provided information for choosing families for in-depth case studies according to a sampling matrix of the following characteristics: caste, socioeconomic status, education, household type (nuclear or joint), and age. This was necessary to capture the variation created by each of these categories. I had to select additional low-caste (or Dalit) families from the two wards for the case studies to compensate for the small number of them in the population. In addition, there were no low-caste families in my random sample that were in the category of moderate or high socioeconomic status.

Ultimately I selected thirty case studies (with two eventually dropping out at different stages in the interview schedule) that represented de facto joint and nuclear families of each caste and, other than the low-caste families, of middle or low socioeconomic status. Wealthy Nepali families were few and anomalous in the area, so I excluded them from the case studies. As mentioned previously, I limited my case study households to Hindu-caste Nepalis—a substantial and influential group, yet only one of many diverse cultural groups found in Nepal.[5] I and my research assistant, Meena, interviewed the married women of reproductive age at each household using a semi-structured, open-ended format an average of five times over the final seven months of my initial research period, and I also had many informal conversations with them along the way.[6] Originally I intended to interview husbands as well, but after discovering a few women were experiencing marital violence I abandoned the idea. The nature of my interviews could have placed women at further risk had I interviewed their husbands. Each interview ranged from thirty minutes to three hours. The topics of interviews were marriage, work, pregnancy, birth and postpartum experiences, and the role of women. The interviews took place alone in the privacy of the women's homes, however some of the most fruitful sessions occurred spontaneously with multiple household members or neighbors present. The first two introductory rounds of household interviews were not taped, but after building rapport I used an audio recorder for the remaining three interviews in the series. Thus all quotes in the book are direct translations of women's recorded statements, the exceptional result of a painstaking process of translation and transcription. A year later, in 2005, I returned for three months of follow-up research with the same case study families. Methods used during the 2009 and 2010 periods of research with young men are described in Chapter four, but I followed up with several of the women from the case studies during those periods as well.

The initial survey I administered in 2003 provides a snapshot of the demographics of the two wards at the beginning of the research period. The average number of years of education was seven for men and four for women. Fifty percent of the families owned their home and the other 50 percent rented. Forty percent of families owned at least one color television. Twenty-one percent owned at least one motorcycle, and 3 percent owned a car. Behind these averages, however, lies diversity. For example, portions of the community were still quite rural and uneducated. In the more urban center of the community, households ranged from joint families who had lived there for generations to unskilled laborers who were new to the area and rented single rooms. At the upper end of the wealth and education spectrum, a handful of families owned a car or had a child with a master's degree. I excluded from the study a few anomalous, considerably wealthy families who owned car companies and international export businesses. At that time, markers of a "middle-class" family typically included a color television, a motorcycle, and possibly a computer. The children in a middle-class family typically would have been educated through the School Leaving Certificate (SLC), with young men having more education on average than young women.

Gender, Caste, and Class

All three of the categories in the title of this chapter—gender, caste, and class—are flawed in that they give the appearance of neat sociological categories that can be applied to societies all around the world. In fact, such categories need to be deconstructed and critiqued, for in different societies they are likely to be defined and lived differently. As Bina Pradhan points out in her summary of the gendered dimensions of development, the concept of gender, for example, is relatively new, and it does not exist as a single word in many languages around the world (2006). Furthermore, Seira Tamang argues that the concept of "Nepali women" only exists because of the way the development industry has construed them as falsely similar (2002).

Such definitions change over time, as well; they are subject to historical forces. Caste, for example, has often mistakenly been seen as a timeless characteristic of the Indian subcontinent. The word caste, in fact, originates in the colonial period from the Portuguese word *castas*, and conflates the Indian *varna*, the ranking system, with *jaati* (*jaat* in Nepali), the cultural and interactional system in practice. Susan Bayly argues that caste must be considered in relation to India's social and political history, particularly the role of colonial powers and independence, and not solely as a feature of a false monolithic and static notion of Hindu ideology (1999). Furthermore, caste is practiced differently all across India. Scholars of India have engaged in a long, rich debate over what caste is and is not and its relationship to a Hindu ideology of purity and pollution versus its function of a system of power and control over people and resources (see Mines 2009 for a summary).

Such a debate has not dominated scholarship or popular imagination of Nepal, however; the politically orchestrated nature of the caste hierarchy is so apparent that there has been much less of a tendency to essentialize it as part of an imaginary Nepalese or Hindu "culture." The caste hierarchy in Nepal resulted from specific historical circumstances including the settlement of a vast variety of cultural and linguistic groups and the eventual political unification of those groups. The Shah dynasty established political (and to a great extent, social and religious) power through conquest of the Kathmandu Valley in 1769, building the Gorkhali kingdom and the foundation of the modern state of Nepal. Subsequently in 1854, the first Rana ruler further attempted to consolidate local and previously independent rulers under a single corpus of laws, the *Muluki Ain*. In a portion of the document, all groups were assigned a status within a single model of hierarchy (see Appendix 1). A wide variety of ethnic groups—some who practiced Hinduism but many who did not—were slotted roughly into a middle position on the hierarchy, below the high castes that observed Hindu practices of abstaining from meat, alcohol, and other ritually polluting substances, and above the "untouchable," low-caste, Dalit groups who engaged in such practices. For over two centuries, law and custom originated from such upper-caste, Parbatiya (hill-dwelling) Hindu rulers. The caste hierarchy was met with various levels of acceptance and rejection, across groups within the hierarchy as well as across regions of the country, with little attention paid in areas remote from the centralized government of the Kathmandu Valley. Historically, the significance of *jaat* (caste/ethnicity/species/kind) in Nepal has changed as well. Since the abolition of discrimination based on caste and the advent of a more inclusive, democratic form of governance, people of the middle and low jaat statuses have attempted to utilize their subjugated position to their advantage politically (Guneratne 2002). Such strategies have intensified with attempts since 2008 at forming a new constitution and the resulting debates over representation and ethnic federalism. And all of the statuses are being re/created in terms of modernity and cultural and linguistic heritage rather than Hindu ideology (Guneratne 2001).

Ideas of purity and pollution are central to discussions of caste and gender in Nepal, as Mary Cameron has argued, and particularly so for groups like the Parbatiya castes of this book who subscribe to rules of impurity avoidance.[7] Therefore it is worth paraphrasing Cameron's summary of these rules at length (1998, 7):

Purity and impurity, or pollution, are concepts found in Hindu cultures that refer to states of people, objects, and actions. Pollution (sometimes called ritual pollution to distinguish it from the Western idea of secular dirt and waste) is of three broad types: that incurred by death, birth, and miscarriage; contact with various objects

(metals, cooking utensils, soiled garments, places, animals); and contact with parts of the body (feet, sex organs) and bodily substances
(saliva, phlegm, semen, blood). Water is a potent transmitter of both
purity and impurity because it is used to purify through bathing
(and an abbreviated form of bathing, sprinkling), but foods impure
people cook in water cannot be eaten by the pure (for example,
uncooked rice, *chaamal*, is neutral, but cooked rice, *bhaat*, is not).
It is in the nature of certain classes of people to possess impurity in
varying degrees, such as women who have bodily impurity and lower
castes that have both bodily impurity and what is called occupational
impurity. Occupational impurity is associated with the lower castes
because they handle materials (metals, leather) and perform acts
(plowing, eating beef) considered impure, and they pass this impure
state onto the next generation. Finally, impurity is temporally bound:
some occupational impurity is temporary, such as plowing, while
other is permanent, such as sewing leather.

In my experience, a wide range of adherence to impurity avoidance existed
among Parbatiya families, to the extent that some families who did not
subscribe to the notion of caste impurity nonetheless adhered to rules
about other forms of impurity, such as women's avoidance of cooking during their menstruation or the *juTho* (polluted) status of used plates and
utensils and, by extension, the kitchen sink.

In sum, seemingly straightforward categories such as gender or caste
are always imbued with power, contested, fluid, and redefined through
practice. Therefore each of these three categories—gender, caste, and
class—will be broken down and investigated as they are practiced in the
daily lives of the women in the following case studies, with particular
attention to the unique ways they intersect. Using a matrix of the possible
combinations of gender, caste, class, and household type (nuclear or multi-
generational), I selected thirty case studies from the 794 households that
I enumerated in the area. Since all of the case studies in this research were
Parbatiya Hindu families from a range of castes, the following discussion
is limited to these three categories and does not address the full range of
dimensions of exclusion present in Nepal, which is nicely summarized by
anthropologist Lynn Bennett and colleagues from the World Bank and
DFID (2006) (See Table 1).

In the sections that follow, four women's stories are arranged according to four caste and class combinations in order to demonstrate how
greatly their life situations are impacted by these social characteristics, and
the patterns of variation that would be lost if one overlooked these inter-
secting forces. The first woman, Ganga, is both high-caste and high-class.

TABLE 1. Dimensions of Exclusion in Nepal

Social Category/ Status	Gender	Caste	Ethnicity/ Race*	Language	Religion	Geo-political
Dominant	Men/ Boys	Brahmin, Chhetri	Caucasoid	Nepali	Hindu	Parbatiya (Hill dweller)
Subordinate	Women/ Girls	Dalit	Janajati/ Mongoloid	Other	Non-Hindu	Madhesi (Plains dweller)

SOURCE: Adapted from "Unequal Citizens" (World Bank and DFID 2006).
*The categories Caucasoid and Mongoloid are highly problematic racial categories, no longer in use. However, in Nepal these terms are still used to differentiate roughly between those groups whose language descends from Indo-European versus Tibeto-Burman prototypes. Susan Hangen (2005) describes how a racial identity of "Mongol" was promulgated in Nepal, in fact, by a collection of ethnic groups to claim a united identity and thereby mobilize political power.

The second, Devi, is high-caste but low in class status. The third woman, Radha, is both low-caste and low in class standing, and the last family is one of the few who is low-caste but high-class. The last family, however, is not a case study at all; their refusal to participate in the study provides an opportunity for a discussion of the significance of the *lack* of a case study for this category.

Ganga (High-Caste, High-Class) (HH #246)

Ganga was 22 years old when I first met her in her large but modest home.[8] I selected her household as one of the case studies because her family was Chhetri, one of the higher castes in the Nepal system, and was of moderately high class standing as well. They would not qualify as wealthy or part of the small elite class of Nepal; they were economically comfortable, but their lives did not include luxuries common among the elite, such as cars, drivers, security guards, cooks, cleaning staff, and gardeners. They were involved in multiple income-generating activities (a small restaurant, overseeing agricultural work and the sale of grains), owned a large, three-storied home, and possessed multiple televisions, motorcycles, computers, and other status markers.

The first time I sat down with Ganga and her mother-in-law, I began interviewing her mother-in-law first out of respect. Soon she was called away to begin cooking food for the restaurant the family owned and operated on the ground floor in the corner of the building, and I never got a chance to interview her again. She was heavily involved in cooking and managing the restaurant. Ganga, in contrast, was always home and willing to chat. During our first hour-long interview, I asked her (as I did for all of the case studies) about her wedding and her transition from her *maaita* (her natal home) to her husband's household, for the dominant marriage settlement pattern for Hindu-caste Nepalis was patrilocal.

Ganga was married when she was fourteen years old. It was an arranged marriage, and she saw and spoke to her husband for the first time at the engagement ceremony. The next time was at the wedding. Ganga's *buDhi saasu* (her mother-in-law's mother-in-law), who was sitting with us during Ganga's interview, estimated that around 1500 guests attended Ganga's wedding. I was amazed by the size. As she shared her wedding photo album with me, I noted the solemn expressions that brides wear, eyes cast downward, during the marriage ceremony. For at marriage, women leave the familiarity of their homes, family relationships, and childhood friends for a household that is unknown to them.

Ganga married after she passed grade seven and was about to start grade eight. After marriage, she did not get the chance to study further. She had the ambition to become a police officer, a strong desire, she said, but was unable to fulfill her wish because she did not get the opportunity to study. She carefully stated that her in-laws did not forbid her to study; however ". . . through marriage they brought a daughter-in-law to work in the house. So who will work in the house, if I go to school the whole day?" Her husband had only studied through grade ten, so studying beyond his level also would have been unsuitable.

Ganga is soft-spoken, quick to smile, and has a calm demeanor. She confided that she felt a little confined within the home of her husband's large joint family. The family did not like for her to go outside, so she rarely left the home even on errands and never left to just walk around (*ghumna jaane*). Four generations of her husband's family lived in the building on the second and third floors. Most of the rooms on the ground floor are rented to several other families, and the small one-room restaurant is in the corner that faces an intersection of two paved roads. Locals often gathered there for a cup of tea, a snack, or a meal during breaks in the agricultural day, or just to chat. Ganga, however, rarely left the top stories of the building, spending most of her time preparing food for the family.

In response to being asked how her husband prefers for her to act, she replied, "He likes me to be simple and not to speak too much and not to speak with men. Some women speak with other men. He used to say, 'Speak with others only when it is necessary and otherwise do not speak.' He does not allow me to go out. There are some people who go for strolls around the village. I don't like to do that. If there is some job to do, I will go; otherwise I will stay at home." Whenever she goes out for some reason, someone from the house always accompanies her. Even when she travels to visit her parents, someone escorts her for her trip there and then fetches her for the return. She does not speak to neighbors, except to call out greetings from the verandah on the roof. "Only greetings like hello. That's all. I don't come down. Other women sit in the street and chat. But I don't come down. I just stay on the kousi." Such behavior is an enactment of high standing in caste and class; "other women" refers to women who work for a living, most likely those who do agricultural work, and perhaps those of ethnic groups or lower castes who do not have the same restrictions on women's mobility or ideals of demure behavior.

When it came to culturally sanctioned activities or trips, such as a woman's return to her natal home (*maaita*) after the birth of a child, Ganga's

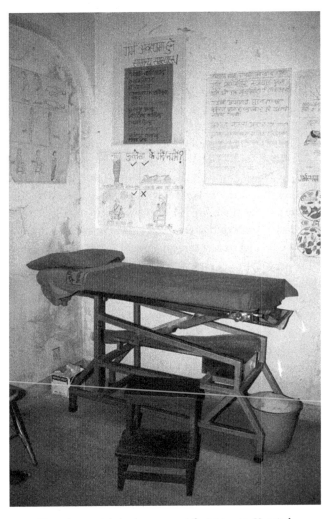

Fig. 5. A prenatal checkup room at the Maternity Hospital.

family was quite accommodating. Both her daughter and son were born by cesarean section at the Teaching Hospital, and both times she was allowed an extended stay of two and a half months at her maita afterwards. During her first pregnancy, they even allowed her to return to her maaita once a month for four or five days at a time. This practice was less common than returning after birth, but her *ghar* (her household/family, which after marriage means her husband's household) assisted her in making these visits. Her husband's family also encouraged her to attend all of her regular prenatal visits at the Teaching Hospital, a ten-minute walk plus a twenty-minute bus ride away, and her mother-in-law went with her. These visits involved standing for several hours in a long line, and Ganga reported that they typically left at 9 A.M. and did not return until 2 P.M. Overall, she said she is lucky because her feelings towards her mother-in-law are similar to those toward her own mother, and her father-in-law is a jovial man who always jokes with the family members. She commented that he always buys and brings fruit as a treat for the women of the household. He always greeted me with a friendly smile and a few polite words when he saw me trudging up and down the mountainside for interviews, something no other man from any of the case studies did.

Overall, Ganga's ghar appeared to be a comfortable domestic setting with an interesting combination of caring gestures towards her, including greater than average freedom to visit her maaita, and some restrictions on her mobility that were typical of a young daughter-in-law of her caste and class status. Typically a greater concern with ritual purity and honor among high castes leads to more restrictions being placed upon high-caste women. Although married couples in general are more prone to polluting behaviors as they must procreate and are often involved in agriculture or artisanal production during the householder stage of life (Cameron 1998), much of the ritual purity of a household falls on the shoulders of its women. Women have a greater risk of polluting a household because of the bodily substances associated with menstruation and birth. Some groups consider women's bodies to be more open/less bounded in general, and thus a better conduit for pollution (Lamb 2000). For these reasons, it follows logically that high castes would need more rules to regulate women's bodies and their behavior in order to maintain a ritually pure and respectable household. Thus caste has had a significant effect on women's gender roles, with restrictions on women's autonomy generally increasing as one moves up the caste hierarchy.

Ganga is a Chhetri woman by birth, so according to the Nepal caste hierarchy she is not a member of the highest group, the Brahmin.[9] Why did I select her, and not a Brahmin, to represent a high-caste, high-class woman? In practice, I discovered that most of the time community members collapsed caste distinctions into two basic categories of high and low. While the Parbatiya Hindu-caste inhabitants of Vishnupura identified themselves in three major high-caste groups, Brahmin or Bahun, Thakuri, and Chhetri, and a multitude of low-caste groups that were once related to occupation, the most common distinction among Parbatiya jaat that I heard local villagers articulate was between small/insignificant (*saano jaat*) and big/important (*Thulo jaat*). And while I heard a couple of educated Thakuri and Brahmin men draw a small number of fine distinctions between the practices of their respective groups in behavior and speech, most people spoke in much more general terms of *saano* or *Thulo*, which I render as low and high in this text for the sake of clarity. I did not dispense with the full list of jaat categories in the research design because I did not want to gloss over any distinctions that might appear, but in the end, it seemed that only high versus low mattered in most everyday discussions and interactions. One exception was that Brahmins were often the subject of jokes about the caste restrictions they followed, or, rather, *failed* to follow—particularly the prohibitions of drinking alcohol and eating meat. Members of other jaats enjoyed teasing Brahmins because of their supposedly superior position at the top of the hierarchy.

Devi (High-Caste, Low-Class) (HH #248)

Another high-caste family selected as a case study happened to live on the ground floor of Ganga's home. High-caste families typically prefer to rent rooms on the bottom floors of their homes to other high-caste families. Devi and her husband were Brahmin. They were renting two rooms and shared a common bathroom with other ground floor tenants. The two rooms consisted of a kitchen and a room with several wooden platform beds, where Devi, her husband, her two boys, and her daughter all slept. Their clean clothes lay in piles on the beds out of lack of space for storage. And as was typical for many of our interviews, we all sat on the beds while we talked. In many homes, firm beds serve as platforms to sit, do homework, play, drink tea, and countless other tasks if the household does not have space for chairs or a separate sitting room. Though the building was well kept, their crowded living conditions and overall economic situation existed in stark contrast with Ganga's multi-generational family just upstairs.

In contrast to Ganga, Devi, a few years older, was rarely home. Devi worked as an informal agricultural laborer in order to pay for food and clothing for her family. Her husband was a teacher at a primary school, but his income was not enough to support even their meager existence.

The only times she was at home were dawn and again in the evenings, often after dark. Before we learned this, we arrived once or twice at different points in the day to try to speak with her. One day we found her eldest son, thirteen at that time in 2003, cooking rice and a vegetable curry for the family's meal (and not simply an easily prepared snack such as instant noodles). His younger brother was assisting him. This sight surprised us, given that sons are not taught to cook unless they show a particular interest. Other than in a restaurant setting, cooking was not generally considered a suitable task for males. Devi had taught her sons how to cook because of her regular absence at meal times.

Devi was accustomed to such long hours of agricultural work from her childhood, so her transition from childhood to married life was not a difficult one. She was raised in a rural village near Panauti, in the hill region east of Kathmandu. She had no formal education. Reflecting on that time, she said,

> I was a small child, thirteen years old, when they came to ask for me in marriage. I don't remember that time. They came to my maaita, and I went to cut fodder carrying the *Doko* (large woven bamboo basket carried on the back with a weight-bearing strap across the forehead). They (her parents) agreed to give me away . . . We (she and her future husband) didn't speak. We also didn't speak for two, three months after marriage. We spoke properly to one another after giving birth to this eldest son.

She had not begun menstruating at the time of her marriage. "The tradition was like that; marriage should be done prior to the start of menstruation." A daughter's sexual purity is of utmost concern to parents, particularly high-caste parents (this will be discussed further in Chapter two). I should note that "speaking" can refer to a variety of interactions in Nepal, from simply speaking briefly or politely, to speaking intimately with someone you know well, and even flirting. Kathryn March writes that "speaking" was even used as a euphemism for sex among the Tamang women with whom she worked (2002, 212). As it is used in the above quote, it likely means to speak freely in a friendly, informal, and therefore intimate way.

Devi's first pregnancy did not occur until several years later when she was eighteen. Her first and subsequent births occurred at home. At the time of her first birth, she was living in her husband's joint family home and worked all day and then went to sleep after eating dinner. She awoke in the middle of the night with labor pains, and while her husband slept she went downstairs to give birth. Her labor lasted only a few hours, and she gave birth alone on the ground floor of the mud house at 3 o'clock in the morning. She did not call out for her mother-in-law, for she was elderly and had rheumatism, and her limbs did not function properly. Devi went to her maaita briefly after the baby was born, but only for nine or ten days because there was no one to do the work in her ghar. They owned a cow and water buffalo, and daily she had to cut fodder for them, clean up the dung, and milk them. I asked what kind of work it was, in comparison, to give birth, to raise, and to care for a young child. Was it very difficult or easy compared to such labor in the fields and with livestock? She replied, "How can it be difficult? I was too busy caring for livestock to care for the baby. So how can caring for a baby be difficult when one cannot do it?" She continued, "There was no time for caring for the baby because I had to do other work."

Devi later described how she had to leave her son alone in a *kokro* (a cradle-like basket suspended from the rafters or a door frame) while she worked, allowing him to sleep, play, defecate, and urinate in the basket, returning only to feed him three times a day. She admitted her children to school as early as possible in order to allow her to work. The second and third children were born after she and her husband moved to Vishnupura. Since her husband worked at a primary school, they were able to admit all the children at no cost as soon as they were old enough to attend. She said, "All were admitted free of charge. Otherwise how could we be able spend lots of money to admit all three children? We depend on earning daily wages in order to eat."

The economic necessity for Devi to work outside of the home set in motion a series of consequences that disrupted gender roles and restrictions for high-caste women. First, allowing her boys to shoulder some of the responsibility of food preparation signifies the dismissal of one of the most symbolic and time-consuming responsibilities for women, cooking for the family. (Her eldest son, thirteen years old when I first met him in 2003, is one of the young men who I interviewed six years later in 2009 when he was nineteen—see Chapter four). Second, her work for various local land-holding families required that she be highly mobile and interact with men and women from the community and those nearby. She occasionally travelled to nearby villages when news spread that they needed extra hands for planting or harvesting. Although she may have taken care to maintain a sense of modesty throughout such interactions, Devi's mobility and public presence challenged the traditional gender expectations for women so readily visible in the behavior of the Chettri family upstairs.

Although many of the differences in gender restrictions were diminished between women like Devi and low-caste women, caste differences were not erased during women's interactions in the agricultural fields in times of work and rest. I heard that it was common for women to separate themselves into smaller groups during breaks to eat meals, and one story was relayed to me in 2005 of a high-caste woman complaining loudly when she was handed a communal water vessel after a low-caste woman had drank from it. This was in spite of the universal, second-nature practice of not allowing one's lips or mouth to touch a water bottle or vessel shared by two or more individuals to prevent making the water—a particularly powerful conveyor of ritual pollution—*juTho* (ritually polluted). Through such performances, women may work to produce difference in situations that otherwise would give the appearance of equals working side by side. Though both low-caste and high-caste agricultural laborers needed the income, sometimes high-caste individuals attempted to establish superiority along a ritual hierarchy to compensate for similar status on a class or economic hierarchy.

Radha (Low-Caste, Low-Class) (HH #483)

Radha, her husband, and her ten-year-old daughter lived in a one-room rental made of unfinished brick near the bazaar. Her family shared an outdoor water tap and outhouse toilet with other renters living in the same one-story structure with a tin roof. The structure was located behind the landlord's four-story home, with a footpath that led to the main street. The list of straightforward questions I had constructed turned out to evoke particularly complex responses in her case, necessitating the telling and retelling of her experiences, because she had led a complicated life despite only being twenty-four. In the first telling certain facts were left out, but the gaps and the numbers that did not add up were left in plain sight. She did not attempt to hide anything about her life, but stylistically it would have seemed rude to announce her circumstances so plainly in the first telling. She seemed to invite us to ask follow-up questions that then elicited the missing details that were key to understanding her life. She would loop back in her storytelling and adjust the narrative. Then once some of those pieces were on the table, she often launched voluntarily into stories that surprised me with their honesty and rawness. As is often the case in anthropological research, it was obvious that in these interactions the anthropologist was hardly perceived as a prying intrusion; on the contrary, Radha was grateful to be heard.

Radha and her husband grew up together in Vishnupura, for they were similar in age. Although in the first go-around she simply said she had had an arranged marriage, gradually important details emerged as we talked. When she was fourteen, she and her soon-to-be husband desired to marry, and they were officially engaged by their respective relatives and attempted to arrange a marriage ceremony jointly with her older sister. However, one of their own relatives interceded and filed a police report to stop them because Radha and her husband were underage. They decided to run off together and elope, and when they returned home the marriage was consecrated by a ceremony in front of relatives in which the groom sprinkles *sindur* in the part of the bride's hair. Then, finally, the last important detail came out—the fact that she was four months pregnant when they eloped. Radha said, "I gave birth to her at the age of fifteen, and people said that a child has given birth to a child." Meena adeptly responded to this revelation by saying that many other women in our interviews had married much younger than she had.

I have written about Radha's relationship with her husband elsewhere (Brunson 2011) and in Chapter three because it figured centrally in her life. Here, however, her employment and mobility are most relevant to the discussion of the ways caste, class, and gender intersect. The nature of Radha's employment stood out from that of the other low-caste women in the case studies, for all the other women were engaged in entrepreneurial work near or in their homes, such as tailoring or operating a fruit stand. Radha worked as a janitor at a hospital, which required much independent mobility on her part as she took the bus to and from work. Moreover, she worked the evening shift. Not only was she regularly travelling alone on public transportation, she was also doing so at night. Travelling alone at night was unheard of for women in this area, including the foreign anthropologist. As a result, people gossiped about the possibility of her being a prostitute. Her husband and father-in-law did not like this aspect of her work, but according to Radha her husband was fiercely independent and spent much time and money on entertainment outside of the house, including food, alcohol, and, she suspected, other women. Sometimes he left for a few days at a time. He wanted her to work and earn so that he did not have to provide everything for her. She felt she needed her own income because occasionally he was unable to provide food or even the money for rent.

Do Radha's wage-earning job and her freedom of movement mean that she has more autonomy than high-caste women? In her study of gender and caste in far western Nepal in the late 1980s, Cameron investigated the experiences and perspectives of low-caste women in order to articulate the ways their lives differed from the dominant discourse on gender and high-caste women. She demonstrated that although low-caste women are ritually impure according to the high-caste perspective, a different set of ideals superseded the purity/pollution ideology of caste for low-caste women. Their contribution to subsistence and wage-earning activities allowed them a social autonomy and relative economic power that most high-caste women did not have. The economic necessity for women to be engaged in labor related to agricultural work or other small-scale earning activities ultimately freed them from some of the patriarchal restrictions on mobility and interactions outside of the home. While Cameron concluded that low-caste women's income and the social benefits of their labor give them more leverage than upper-caste women who depend on honor for their ideological power, she argued for a more nuanced reading of low-caste women's autonomy than the simple claim that low-caste women have more freedom and autonomy than women of high caste (Cameron 1998).

Radha's story provides some of this nuance. As a low-caste woman, she does indeed have the freedom to work outside the home, be mobile, interact on her own terms with neighbors and community members, and engage with the public through her job. These characteristics held true for the other four low-caste women in the case studies, as well, other than the fact that they worked very near to where they lived. These distinctions in autonomy are recognized by low- and high-caste alike. One high-caste woman commented, "People say that the life of lower caste women is freer than the life of higher caste women. For example, the lower caste can do any job and go anywhere." Overall, the experiences of low-caste, low-class women in Vishnupura bear out Cameron's findings on low-caste women's rejection of high-caste gender rules. In these families, women did not have to show as much deference to their husbands through respectful forms of speech and behavior. All were engaged in income-generating activities. Three women worked as tailors in self- or family-owned businesses and operated one-room shops. They managed all aspects of the businesses: taking orders, sewing, and negotiating prices. A fourth, destitute woman managed her own fruit shop, selling whatever was in season at her road-side stall. She handled all management aspects of the small business, often travelling an hour's distance by bus to the wholesale market where she purchased her fruit, and setting and negotiating her prices according to various market influences.

Despite such autonomy, Radha experienced a significant backlash to her independent movements from the larger community. While wage-earning or entrepreneurial work and mobility were the norm for low-caste women, and part of the accepted gender role, other community members spoke against her moral character and gossiped that she was a prostitute. In the views and reactions of the larger community, Radha had transgressed the dominant (i.e. high-caste) perspective on gender roles. These public expressions of disapproval seem to indicate that she in fact should not be working and moving about in this fashion. Thus to say that low-caste women are exempt from the gender rules of the dominant high castes is to miss this matter of clash in perspectives and the disapproval that is expressed from the larger community or society. One young, low-caste woman who worked as a tailor said, "Society wants a woman to stay inside the house and not speak with anyone, otherwise they start backbiting you. Even if we wear nice clothing, they will talk about us and start commenting that so-and-so's daughter-in-law is behaving like this and that. We can't speak with outsiders." Such a statement sounds like it should have been spoken by a high-caste woman. Going out, wearing (and thus flaunting) nice clothing, and conversing freely with non-family members are all described as acts of immodesty that may bring social scorn upon a woman. The difference in the experience of gender for low-caste women in Vishnupura, then, is their attempt to reject the dominant society's gender roles while, at the same time, they are looked down upon for doing so by the dominant society. Effectively they operate in dual systems of gender, for they cannot escape the dominant high-caste society's perspective. While acting according to one system of gender, they face potential repercussions from another.

The Family Who Refused (Low-Caste, High-Class)

Devi's case, along with the other high-caste women who worked out of necessity to support their families economically, suggests that impoverishment trumps high caste status when it comes to following gender norms for women. In practice, many of the gender restrictions typically placed on high-caste women's behavior were loosened considerably, or ignored, in the face of the need to earn an income. Consider the other possibility; does being wealthy trump one's low-caste status? Do wealthy, low-caste women find themselves subject to the gender restrictions of high-caste women, and thus lose some of their stereotypical freedoms? I cannot answer this question based on my fieldwork, but an explanation of the reasons why I cannot answer it is itself instructive.

The Sarki family is a local family, with their residence in Vishnupura going back several generations.[10] They live in a large, two-story home on a quiet side street a small distance up the mountain and away from the chaotic bazaar. A magenta bougainvillea grows up the large wall and across the cast-iron gate that protect the compound from unannounced visitors, but the small guard house by the gate was always empty. The joint family's motorcycles and car were usually parked in the concrete driveway inside the gate. They owned a small shoe factory on the main road that runs up the mountainside in Vishnupura. From the debris outside the factory on the side of the road, it looked as if they manufactured mostly black rubber flip-flops.

The Sarki family had not been a part of my initial survey of a random sample of 248 households in Wards 1 and 2 in Vishnupura. In that random sample, not a single low-caste family was of high economic status.

There were several low-caste families of modest economic means. There was also an abundance of families who owned land and homes, and several wealthy families who owned cars and employed multiple domestic workers and staff. But there were no low-caste families who owned land, houses, or cars or other such markers of a higher class. Given that this was a statistically significant random sample of all the households in Wards 1 and 2 (I enumerated all of them, N = 794, n = 248), one can conclude that there were very few families like the Sarkis. I sought out such a household to supplement the case studies selected directly from the survey respondents so that this important subgroup of low-caste, high-class households would not be missed. Manoj, my other research assistant whose family home was in Vishnupura, suggested that we talk to the Sarkis because he was an acquaintance of one of the sons, and they were the only family he knew that fit the criteria. Despite this amicable introduction to the family, the Sarkis refused to participate in my research without much explanation. The general impression they gave was that they did not want to be scrutinized; whether they meant by me in my publications or by community members as a result of participating in the research—or both—was unclear.

Laura Ahearn (2001a) and Cameron (1998) relay stories of footholds Dalits gained in the 1990s in villages in western Nepal in respect to ritual and economic domains, as well as the limits that they encountered, and Andrea Nightingale (2011) provides a few more recent examples of the production of difference between high-caste and Dalits in rural northwestern Nepal. However, the stories of wealthy Dalit women are absent from the scholarly literature on Nepal. Comparable to the way that Radha was criticized by the wider society even though she was not breaking the gender norms of her own relatives and caste, it may be the case that low-caste, wealthy women find themselves subject to even greater scrutiny by the dominant members of the wider community and society. While I can conclude through multiple examples that the necessity to engage in income-generating labor trumps high caste status and related gender expectations, I suspect that being wealthy does not free low-caste individuals of discrimination based on caste and might, in fact, lead to decreased autonomy and greater public scrutiny for low-caste women in particular.

Conclusion

These examples of the ways that caste, class, and gender intersect defy generalizations based on any one single category. Combining theoretical advances on gender and intersectionality made by scholars like Kimberle Crenshaw in the United States (1989; 1991) and Chandra Mohanty in respect to the global South (1984; 2003), with discussions of caste and class in scholarship on Nepal cited above, my theoretical contributions in this chapter to understanding the meanings, practice, and lived experience of these categories in Nepal are threefold.

First, I suggest that poverty acts as a leveling mechanism between low-caste and high-caste women, making it impossible for either to live by the dominant set of high-caste gender ideals. However, as the example of objections to sharing a water vessel in a rice field showed, small acts of maintaining or reestablishing a ritual hierarchy based on notions of jaat may still be enacted under these conditions. Thus at least in the case of economically disadvantaged families, women may attempt to employ their higher caste status to maintain a higher social standing on at least one of the axes of identity.

Second, I ask what are the implications of arguing that poor high- and low-caste women have more autonomy, while as a result of their poverty, they engage in physically demanding labor (in the case of agricultural or construction work) or have difficulty purchasing and consuming nutritious foods or obtaining health care (applicable more broadly, even for those involved in small-scale entrepreneurial work)? To consider autonomy as a primary indicator of women's well-being would be to miss the effects of poverty on women's overall health and fulfillment. When talking about women's autonomy, other measures of discrepancies in power according to one's position in multiple hierarchies of social status must also be invoked, and attention paid to how they interact (Brunson 2013). The effects of poverty can too easily be misinterpreted and dismissed as a result of "culture" by outsiders, particularly when it comes to matters of well-being (Farmer 1999), or naturalized by insiders as a result of a subgroup's cosmic "place," racialized "nature," or "backward" status (Cameron 1998; Guneratne 2001; Pigg 1992). In order to adequately address the relationship between women, power, and health, in-depth anthropological research is needed. Rather than viewing variation at the individual level as something that needs to be smoothed over through larger samples and bell curves, I argue that in-depth qualitative research enables the instructive nature of such examples to be revealed. Statistical analysis alone would erase the humanity of women such as the ones portrayed here, along with the distinctive configurations of domination or suffering they experience because of how intersectionality operates in their lives.[11]

My third contribution is a modest one—simply to expose the lacuna in the anthropological literature regarding the gendered experiences of low-caste, wealthy women in Nepal. As financial opportunities slowly begin to open for Dalit families in a nascent democratic, capitalist, secular system, how do old forms of discrimination transform in economic centers like the Kathmandu Valley? And how are these experiences different for Dalit men and women? What are the new structural opportunities and constraints for success for Dalit women, and what social norms influence their identities?

The meanings of caste and ethnicity are always in flux in Nepal, and the major political and social developments that have been occurring during and since this research was completed in 2010 have had significant impacts on the ways that Nepalis are self-identifying and defining one another (see Hangen 2010; Lawoti and Hangen 2013; Mishra and Gurung 2012). The conclusion of the Maoist People's War in 2006, which had aimed to end the monarchy and abolish other social inequities of caste, class, and gender, led to serious public discussions and challenges to long-standing religious, caste, ethnic, gender, geographic, and linguistic hierarchies in Nepal. The election of the Constituent Assembly and attempts to write a new constitution have also contributed toward the development of cultural identity-based movements, with many of these identities taking shape during and post conflict (World Bank and DFID 2006). These emergent identities along with the gradual unseating of historically dominant groups have the potential to create new configurations of identity and dominance (or equity) in Nepal. But as of 2010, many mainstream Nepalis in the Kathmandu Valley opined that while the significance of caste was fading, much remained the same in post-monarchy Nepal. I will return to this situation in Chapter four.

To conclude, in this chapter I tackled the challenge of analyzing culture and inequality and the embodied experience of social hierarchy among Hindu-caste Nepali women. I addressed, in very human terms, a range of structural components of Nepali society that motivate and constrain women's agency. I began by exploring the ways that caste and class intersect with gender norms and divide or reconfigure women's experiences, and I argue that poverty has the power to diminish these moral systems of hierarchy in specific ways.

In the pages that follow, I further complicate an understanding of women's experience of gender by taking a life course perspective and demonstrating with illustrations at the micro level the significant changes in status that occur over a lifetime in culturally determined ways. After revealing and accounting for the complexity and interaction of these layers of social hierarchy and historical change, I turn to the experience of procreation. I argue that women engage in complex projects of reproduction that reveal both the structural constraints placed upon them by local and global discourses as well as the potential for creativity in their responses.

2

Like a Potter's Wheel

From Daughters to Mothers-in-Law

In addition to caste and class, as illustrated in the last chapter, a woman's stage of life significantly impacts her position and relative power vis-à-vis other family members and the number and severity of gender restrictions. While the last chapter considered social hierarchies, this chapter focuses on familial hierarchies and the life course. My observations of families constitute a limited slice of family life, with different members located in different positions, for example, a new wife, a wife with young children, or a mother-in-law. My retrospective interviews with women, however, allowed me to capture an additional perspective as women reviewed their progression through the relevant stages of the life course. Many women talked about female life course stages as a timeless cycle, one family comparing it to a potter's wheel. I also asked women to speculate on the experience of moving into the next stage of life, for example what would it be like to become a mother-in-law instead of a daughter-in-law? And I inquired about differences between their experiences and the experiences of their daughters. The retrospective and "imagine the future" parts of the interviews successfully elicited the kinds of changes women observed over time, making it undeniable that life course stages are not part of a fixed, ahistorical cycle. In this way, although the cyclical potter's wheel trope may capture women's portrayals of their circulation out of and into households over the generations, the shortcomings of this metaphor are apparent and instructive.

The dominant family system among Hindu-caste Nepalis, along with much of Hindu South Asia, is the multi-generational joint family, with patrilocal marriage practices and patrilineal inheritance and kinship. This does not mean that all families are in fact joint families at any one point in time. Tom Fricke's research, for example, conducted with a Tamang community not far from my research site, exhibited in detail the cycle of joint families and how married sons split off from the stem family when the number of family members becomes too great for maintaining harmony and sharing resources as a single unit (Fricke 1994). Thus a number of families will always be in a nuclear stage within a joint family system (see Skinner 1997), and detecting a trend towards a conjugal family system is tricky. It would take another generation or two to determine whether the nuclear families in my study would remain nuclear. More important for this study, in the end, was their belief that they would become joint families again (Brunson 2010).

Within a multi-generational joint family system, life course stages are typically particularly salient for women, as their status changes dramatically with marriage, the birth of children, and the marriage of those children. In the dominant ideal for a Hindu Nepali woman, she moves from being considered the embodiment of the goddess as a young daughter, innocent and pure, to a sexual being who is simultaneously a threat to her husband's patriline and the vital source of its continuation (Bennett 1982). Finally she becomes considered an asexual, post-menopausal being with few gender restrictions (Das 1992; Lamb 2000). During the married reproductive years, women's positions vary dramatically within the household family system. Historically within much of Nepal and northern India, the predominant pattern of marital residence has been patrilocal with multi-generational extended family living arrangements (Fruzzetti 1982; Fruzzetti et al. 1992; Vatuk 1975). In this system, the new wife bears the greatest burden of domestic duties and has the lowest status in the hierarchy of the family. Over time, her position improves as she produces children, especially sons, and as other wives are brought into the family by her husband's brothers. Eventually, her status increases considerably when her son brings a new wife into the household (Das Gupta 1995). Monica Das Gupta (1995) has demonstrated that in northern India, an area somewhat culturally similar to middle and southern Nepal, fertility preferences and maternal and child health differ dramatically according to the life course status of the woman and the sex of her children, when controlling for established predictors such as education, wealth, and caste.

In sum, one's life stage evolves, households themselves are dynamic, and history is always unfolding and interacting with both. Thus women's power and the gender restrictions they face are always in flux. This, in turn, impacts demographic outcomes for women such as health and fertility. Das Gupta's description of the north Indian joint family system and its impact on women's health is germane to the Hindu groups with which I was working in Nepal as well:

> there are strong intergenerational and intragenerational bonds between household members related to each other by blood. Concomitantly, the development of a strong conjugal bond is discouraged. This means that the woman marrying into the household is in a very weak position in terms of making decisions to protect her own and her children's health. Layers of people are above her in the household hierarchy of status and authority, beginning with all the adult males, and continuing through all the women older than her (1997, 43).

While such a generalization about women's status and health held true for the Hindu-caste families in Vishnupura, challenges to this familial hierarchy were developing as well. Vishnupura was undergoing a transition from an agricultural to a cash-based economy, and community members were shifting from a familial mode of production to a non-familial mode of organization of life's fundamental activities (see Axinn 1992; Axinn and Yabiku 2001) or a capitalist mode of production. Among other things, this meant that more young men and women were attending school longer, despite the fact that actual opportunities for employment had not caught up with the increase in the value of education and the number of educated workers. Increases in the education of girls resulted in scenarios in households where daughters-in-law were significantly more educated than mothers-in-law. Such changes undermined the traditional familial hierarchy and were the subject of much intergenerational joking and teasing.

Life as a Daughter, Labor as a Daughter-in-Law, Uncertainty as a Mother-in-Law

In Lynn Bennett's classic ethnography on high-caste Hindu groups in Nepal, she argues that symbolically women are not fully members either in their natal or marital homes (1982). Being a daughter is like being a guest in a household that provides care and nourishment, for a daughter will inevitably leave the household and her consanguineal kin. As a child, a daughter is cherished as an embodiment of the goddess, as a pure being. Although the protection of her purity is a major duty of her parents, a daughter is fairly free within the confines of her home to do things like speak her mind and wear comfortable and casual clothing. She is not responsible for the future of her natal family through progeny, name, wealth, or success. And though the laws have changed to allow women to inherit land, in practice inheritance and name are passed down mostly through men.

For women, marriage represents a physical separation from people and place, but also a symbolic shift in points of reference in the most intimate and fundamental of ways: a redefining of self, family, and home. That such changes come with marriage is not unique to Nepal, but the ways these transformations take place are context-specific and consequentially have particular outcomes in terms of women's autonomy, health, and fertility. As a wife, a woman is symbolically responsible for producing the descendants of her husband's family and protecting its good name through her piety and devotion. Her claim to the family name, though, remains an indirect one—it operates through her husband. In the case of early widowhood or separation, a woman's affines may easily shirk even the most basic responsibilities toward the woman, such as shelter and food (see Van Hollen 2013). Even women's inheritance from consanguineal kin given to her at the time of marriage (*daijo*) is often forfeited should a woman ever seek the rare option of leaving or divorcing a man (Weiss 1999). Thus one could argue that a woman is never truly at home in the home of her husband, or in the case of old age, her son.

In order to portray the fundamental commonalities and the potential for uniqueness in women's experiences of the transition from daughter to daughter-in-law, I provide one woman's detailed story of becoming a bride, a daughter-in-law, a mother, and her thoughts on becoming a mother-in-law. Her story begins each of the following sections on these topics. Focusing on Maya's (HH #140) life history in some detail provides a much more poignant and human explanation of social processes and avoids the undesirable objectification and distancing that so easily occurs in social science writing. It also creates a structure for examining the most relevant points common to many of the women in this study.[1] When I first interviewed Maya, she was 37 years old and had two daughters and one son. Her eldest daughter was studying for a college degree and working part time as a teacher. Her husband had a salaried job, and the family was middle-class and of the Chettri *jaat*. They had few outward markers of the middle class; they lived in a modest brick and cement house on a small, narrow plot of land, and they still owned some agricultural land some distance away. In the segments of her story, I try to preserve the language that Maya used in telling it, though I use the third person since I am summarizing rather than using direct quotes. I occasionally break into the narrative with her exact words for emphasis or when an English equivalent does not do justice to the meaning of the original Nepali words or expressions.

A Daughter Becomes a Bride

Maya met her husband for the first time on her wedding day. At first her mother had said that she did not want to give her daughter to anyone who lived in Vishnupura. The place was not "developed" (*bikaasi*) at all at that time; it was merely a small village. After seeing her future son-in-law, however, she changed her mind. She liked him.

Representatives from the prospective groom's side and from Maya's side met at the groom's house. At first her mother had said that Maya should not be given away to such a place, but her relatives recommended that she go to see what it was like. Reluctantly her mother went to the boy's house, saying that she would go only as a formality. But after seeing the boy, on the way back home, she felt that he would take care of (*paalchha*) her daughter.

Maya's prospective husband had six brothers; despite that being the case, her mother decided to give her to one of them. This meant that their property would be divided among the seven brothers, and each one's piece would be small. Maya's mother began planning to give her away in marriage, and she informed Maya. Soon *phupaaju* (Maya's uncle) and *bhinaaju* (her brother-in-law) went, gave *Tikaa*, and left. "It's like this for us, our tradition—give *Tikaa* to the boy, fix the details of the wedding, give *janai* (sacred thread) and *supaari* (betel nut), and 'From today we have given our daughter to you' has to be said by the mother to the future husband."

At that time (around 1983), people did not meet before the wedding. Some people probably did, but she and her two sisters definitely did not. The wedding happened "all at once" (*ekai choTi*). No one from the husband's side came to Maya's house to arrange the marriage, but Maya's was an unusual case. She had no brothers, only sisters, and her father had passed away while she was still in her mother's womb. Seven months after his death, she was born. Her father had spent all the inheritance before passing away, and Maya and her mother stayed there in the village until she got married. After she left her village, Maya's mother lived with Maya's older sister's family (for her mother had no sons).

For the wedding day, they called all of the villagers in Maya's village. A busload of guests had arrived from the groom's side, in addition to around thirty local wedding guests. There were only fifteen or sixteen houses in her village at that time. She had not fixed her makeup or hair when the *janti* (groom's procession) arrived. She was sitting outside, just like that. And then someone said, "Well, the groom has already been brought and you haven't done your makeup!" Then friends came to arrange her hair for her, and her mother told her to put on everything. And her mother asked if she needed any assistance to arrange her hair. They put on makeup, the wedding occurred, and in the evening they took her. She returned with the guests, musicians, and everyone in that bus. They reached there around eight o'clock at night and had to walk after the road ended. She had had only a glass or two of water. They said to feed her, but she did not feel like eating. It was a different kind of food than she was accustomed to at her old home, and she wondered how she could survive eating such food. It was very uncomfortable for her. Leaving her own home was difficult. One does not know what it will be like. She was seventeen when she got married; it was not so early. Despite that, she cried.

"Why wouldn't one cry? Leaving one's own home and going to another, won't a person cry then?!" Before the wedding there had been only the two of them living together, mother and daughter. Whenever Maya went out, her mother used to wait for her to return until she made tea. Her mother always used to wait for her before eating anything. After giving *Tikaa* to Maya's future husband, her mother did not cry in front of her, but behind her back she cried loudly—every day after fixing the date of the wedding. Thinking that Maya would hear, her mother would go to the garden to cry. In one place Maya would cry, and in another place her mother would cry, separately.

Daughters in Nepali Hindu families are shielded by their mothers from the harsher aspects of life as a woman, including work. Daughters have responsibilities in the household from an early age, sometimes from age six or seven, but children are mostly indulged before that. Young daughters learn to wash the metal plates and cups, wash clothes, and shadow their mothers in the kitchen. For the most part they are not asked to do physically demanding work. This is contingent upon the socio-economic standing of the family; in very poor families children must shoulder, often literally, much physical work. Destitute young boys are even employed outside the home in the informal economy in positions such as fare collectors on public transportation.

Daughters help out in household work, and they are chided if they do not or if they act "lazy;" but as Maya said in the part of her story that follows, daughters have the option of saying "I can't." This important distinction applies to a range of situations, including becoming tired from work, not knowing how to do a particular job, or having a competing obligation. I observed numerous situations in which adolescent daughters who had an important test coming up in school were able to skip their normal household duties. Alternatively, if agricultural work such as carrying heavy sacks of rice or planting is too difficult, girls can decline. This is increasingly true with the changes in ideals among the middle class. The involvement of young people in agricultural work is increasingly looked down upon by those who have the financial means to avoid it.

In the end, girls are not responsible for making sure the work gets done and the household runs smoothly—that responsibility falls on the mother/daughter-in-law. In fact, the differences between the status of a daughter and a daughter-in-law are the most palpable in the differential standing of two women in a single multi-generational family. In a situation where there are unmarried daughters still living at home with a son, his wife, and his parents, the daughters in the family have very few responsibilities or concerns because they are all handed over to the daughter-in-law. In several situations of this kind, the daughter-in-law seemed more like a hired domestic worker in the home than a family member. The daughter-in-law adopted behavior like not speaking and looking at the ground when in the presence of a daughter in the family. And countless times I overheard daughters yelling for the daughter-in-law of the house, calling her loudly by her kin name, "*Bhaauju!*" and yelling orders that permeated the rooms of the house to bring tea, fix snacks, or locate this or that missing object.

Maya's description of her mother waiting until Maya arrived home to drink tea and eat with her is indicative of the special treatment women receive while their main identity is that of a daughter. Food and eating are highly symbolic in Hindu cultures, and Maya's inclusion of this detail in the story of her life as a daughter would be tacitly meaningful to another Nepali or someone familiar with Hindu cultural symbolism. Food is central in familial and social relationships. In addition to the purity and pollution rules governing food and especially cooked rice that remain widely acknowledged in South Asia, the act of eating and the order in which people eat is of substantial significance. As a general rule, women of the lowest status in the household eat last after serving the other members, although I observed plenty of exceptions to this among the families with whom I was close. On the whole, a daughter-in-law of a joint family would not eat until the other senior members had been served or had finished eating, and the mother in a nuclear family would do the same. I would be remiss to reduce the interpretation of this practice to the oppression of women and the denial of choice foods and nutrition to women—although these outcomes do occur, and they pose particular problems for women who are pregnant or breastfeeding. A more nuanced explanation of this behavior pays attention to women's emotional and strategic reasons for eating last. This is one of a range of behaviors that women use to demonstrate their devotion for their husbands and families. This behavior may be felt genuinely and deeply as an expression of devotion, or it may be acted out as merely a required duty depending on the specifics of a woman's relationships. Overall, feeding someone is a poignant expression of caring for them. And the actual placing of food in someone's mouth, whether by a parent for a child, or by bride and groom in the marriage ritual, is even more highly symbolic. The transgression in these two instances of the *juTho* rules that are typically in place signifies the marked intimacy and closeness of the two individuals involved. Thus when Maya's mother waited to eat with her, it was an expression of her love for her daughter. And when Maya refused to eat on her wedding day, it was more than a matter of unfamiliar food; not eating a meal is a known expression to others of emotional distress.

Rather than a day of celebration and the symbolic joining of two families, the wedding day in Hindu South Asian societies that practice patrilocal marriage has been a day of separating from one family and joining another. A daughter is given to a new family through the ritual of marriage (Fruzzetti 1982). On the day of the wedding, first the groom and his family and friends travel in a lively procession (*janti*) to the house of the bride. The bride's family hosts the wedding rituals and reception dinner. The various stages of the wedding call on the bride and groom to sit passively while gifts are presented, their feet are washed, and a priest recites scriptures and instructs the pair to perform various rituals. While this is happening, brides characteristically sit with downcast eyes and a solemn, if not sad, expression. Rather than following a social script on correct behavior, women explained that they were genuinely sad on the day of their wedding. Ganga, introduced in Chapter one, elaborated, "You feel like crying, and so you have to bow your head . . . it's not tradition, you really feel like crying." Her *buDhi saasu* (her husband's father's mother) added, "Of course you feel like crying—upon leaving your mother and father, you will feel like crying." Almost all of the women in the case studies reported crying during their weddings. Some older women said they did not cry because they were too young at the time of their marriage to understand what was happening. Several women compared getting married at a young age to playing with dolls, getting a chance to play dress-up in fancy clothes. When it came time to leave home, though, they were distraught. "I felt as though we were playing dolls. I was still small. Even after I was brought here [husband's house] I kept telling them that I wanted to go to my own house. I cried when being sent off. I felt, where am I being sent away to?"

Among women who had arranged marriages and were living in joint families, Maya's story of separation at marriage was typical, although details such as her mother's widowhood and her husband's many brothers were unique. And most of the women in the case studies who were living in nuclear families at the time of the study had lived initially in the joint family prior to splitting. The other few women who had "love marriages" experienced a different kind of separation—some were escaping unhappy relationships with family members and were therefore glad to leave, and some were cast out by their families after the knowledge of their relationship with their husband became public.[2]

Added to the separation from family and friends, as well as the loss of familiar surroundings and routines, is the fact that most women in my case studies had never spoken to the groom prior to their wedding day. They may have seen the groom when he came to see the face (*keti herne*) of the bride and finalize the marriage agreement, but never were words exchanged. One woman exclaimed, "How could I speak to a person whom I didn't know? It was not like now; things were different. We used to run away if some stranger tried to talk to us. We were shy. Only now do people talk first and get married." Themes of separation from family and being entrusted to strangers filled women's stories about marriage, especially those who were reflecting on events from ten or fifteen years ago.

Marriage represented a departure from almost everything that was familiar to a girl—the love and protection of her parents, the comfortable spaces that exist within the walls of the home in which she was free from many of the public gender restrictions on behavior and appearance, and her relationship with family members, neighbors, friends, and places in her hometown. The separation and anxiety that women experience at the time of their weddings are parts of a rite of passage into womanhood. Another part of the transition is a dramatic change in social and kinship roles. Almost overnight, women gain all kinds of new responsibilities, many of which are unfamiliar. For an explication of this aspect of learning to be a daughter-in-law, I return to Maya's story.

Learning to Be a Daughter-in-Law

After Maya came here to her new home, there were a lot of problems. Even though Maya's mother had encountered difficulty in life, she had made sure that her children were happy. At her *maaiti ghar* (a woman's natal family, also referred to as *maaita* when referencing the house or location, i.e. natal home), Maya did not have to do that much work. At her new home there were many family members, a lot of livestock, and many fields. Maya was not accustomed to such work, especially carrying a heavy load for a long distance. She began her duties at her new home on the third day after her marriage. She went to the potato fields to work, and she had to carry a *Doko* of compost. (*Doko* is a large basket designed to be carried on one's back, with a strap—*naamlo*—that sits towards the top of one's forehead.) "I was not able to carry it, and two other people helped me carry it. Still they laugh at me saying that three people helped to carry it . . . I couldn't even walk properly from here to there in this steep area while wearing the *naamlo*." It was very difficult for her to start such work suddenly as an adult.

There is much difference between *maaita* and *ghar* (*ghar* means home, but here *ghar* means a woman's husband's home).[3] There are differences in work, food, dress, and going out. "In *maaita* we don't have to work if we can't. We can say to Mother that we can't do it, and that is alright. 'I don't know how,' or 'I won't,' can be said. But here [in the husband's home] that doesn't work. We have to do it even if we don't know how or we are not able [physically] to do it. That is the difference." Everyone else in Maya's ghar could do more work than she could. And that didn't work, of course, in the household. It took a long time for her to wash her clothes, and in the same amount of time others could finish a lot of work. The others in the family did not wash clothes very often. No matter how dirty the clothes became, they kept wearing the same dirty, torn clothes. Maya's different standards for clean clothes became a major point of contention in the family.

There is also a vast difference in the behavior of mother-in-law (*saasu*) and mother, of course. When Maya's mother scolded her, she did not feel bad. When her husband's relatives scolded her, she felt unhappy. It was different with her own relatives.

Marriage marks the end of being a daughter in many ways, although women return to their natal homes occasionally whenever they get the chance. One's *maaita* remains a safe haven for married women especially during socially sanctioned periods of visitation such as *Dasain*, Mother's Day, or after giving birth. After getting married, a daughter's responsibilities and relationship to her natal home are severed for the most part, however, other than these exceptions and the symbolic responsibility of the *Bhaai Tikaa* ritual. *Bhaai Tikaa* is an annual occasion during the celebration of *Dasain* when the woman's relationship to her brother(s) is strengthened. A sister travels to her natal home on that day and offers her brother(s) blessings through a ritual plate of special food items and putting *Tikaa* on his forehead.

With marriage, a woman's allegiance and service switches over to her new family, the patriline of her husband. A woman's main identity thus changes from a daughter (*chhori*) to a daughter-in-law (*buhaari*). This is reflected in how others address a woman: when calling a married woman, younger people in the community commonly address her as "*Bhaauju*," meaning elder brother's wife. Kinship terms always supersede proper names.

A woman's name is not the only referential that changes. That which she has called her ghar her entire life, she refers to after marriage as her *maaiti* ghar, or *maaita* in the short form. A simple translation of ghar is "home" or "household," but its significance is more complex. Only women have a *maaiti* ghar; for men no such thing exists. A man is always a member of his patriline. He does not experience the leaving of one family/home/household and the joining of a new one in the way that women do. If he leaves his parents' household to form a nuclear family household, he might call both residences his ghar if his new home is one he owns and intends to establish permanently, but more likely he will refer to the new home with a range of other words that carry less significance. A man can also use ghar to refer to his birthplace or place of family origin. And last, ghar can refer collectively to the members of one's patriline, usually to the living members of a joint family household, by either men or married women. The difference is that when married women refer to their ghar, they are always referring to their husband's home or the collective members of that home.

When a bride first arrives at her new home, she is often met with special treatment for at least the first day or two. After that, she is introduced to her new responsibilities or sometimes left on her own, guessing and worrying about what she should be doing in the new house. Women talked about a constant uneasiness in their new ghar, which stemmed mostly from the strangeness of the new place and people along with worries that they would not do tasks the "right" way.

Becoming a wife and daughter-in-law brings major changes in terms of a woman's responsibilities, both in type and rigor. Many young women had never been involved in agricultural work before. Planting, harvesting or reaping, hauling loads, and raising animals such as cows, water buffalo, goats, and chickens were especially foreign to those girls coming to Vishnupura from the urban neighborhoods of Kathmandu. In the late 1980s and 1990s when most of the women in my case studies were getting married, Vishnupura was rural and "undeveloped" as described by Maya's mother. When I first visited Vishnupura in 2000, there was a dirt road leading up the mountainside to the village and only a small bazaar near the temple. There was much wide-open space and fields between the homes. When I returned in the spring of 2003, I hardly recognized the area because of all the new buildings and paved road. And in the eleven-month span of my longest consecutive research stint, between the fall of 2003 and the summer of 2004, houses were being built at such a fast rate that the landscape seemed to change almost daily.

Back when many of the women first moved to Vishnupura at the time of their marriage, it was little more than a forest, according to one Brahmin woman originally from Kathmandu. When she first arrived in the village after her wedding, she cried and cried upon seeing the surrounding forest. "There were such big boulders everywhere," she said, "but nowadays nice houses have been built all around, and it's nice now." Gathering firewood in that forest for cooking, undertaking agricultural work, and raising livestock were daunting to the women from urban families. Another woman raised in Kathmandu described the early years of her marriage, during which she had to gather firewood and fodder, saying, "I rarely talk with anyone about this. Thinking about the past, I want to cry; it was so sad. All over (gestured towards arms) there were wounds. I had to go to the forest, and my feet and legs were scratched all over. It used to be like that." Women in farming families work hard in the fields; plowing the earth is the only task restricted to men. Married women of low economic status are forced into positions of paid hard labor such as carrying loads of construction materials or fodder, or doing the most back-breaking parts of farming for land-owning families.

In married women's stories about their pasts as well as my observations of young unmarried women, there was a general desire to move away from agriculture as a source of livelihood. The two women quoted above stressed how much more pleasant their lives had become after they were able to quit doing work like transplanting rice and gathering fodder from the forest. For some families, income from selling land or a wage-paying or salaried job supplanted toil in the fields. Historical developments such as a growing economy and education system made this possible. Improvement in Maya's position was related to her husband obtaining a modest salaried job and leaving the joint family—a major shift in lifestyle. She was able to leave behind arduous agricultural tasks and her share of the duties in a large joint family. Maya attributed their separation from the joint family household mostly to her inability to do the requisite work, but it was her husband's salary that enabled them to start building a new house. In her case it was a combination of economic developments and a change in household structure that precipitated the change in her duties and status.

Becoming a Mother

Maya became pregnant with her first child just shy of two years after her wedding. At that point she and her husband were still living with the joint family. It was during planting season, and she was fed *chiuraa* (beaten rice) and *achaar* (a fresh, cooked, or pickled relish, typically spicy or sour) while working in the rice fields. She didn't eat meals with the family in the early months of pregnancy. "I couldn't find food that I liked in the house, so how could I eat? . . . Sometimes I drank *mahi* (a drink from the liquid strained off from making yogurt) or tea; otherwise I didn't usually eat." When it came time to give birth, her labor lasted five days. "And after not being able to eat for five days, one vomits, of course. Whatever was eaten was vomited. From Wednesday to Friday. And on Saturday, after vomiting and vomiting, there was blood in the vomit. At that time my husband said it wasn't good to keep me at home . . . On Saturday morning around noon they took me to Thapathali Hospital, and my daughter was born Sunday morning."

"And, without eating anything, and having a strong fever, I was just like a crazy person . . . for four to five days I didn't know where or what or anything." She returned home after six days in the hospital.

After eighteen days, Maya went to her *maaita* to rest while recovering from birth. She stayed with her mother for around one month, and then her husband was granted permission to move out of the joint family home. Her husband came to get her, and she returned to their new house with him and her mother. "It was a newly built house; there weren't any windows or doors, only the main door. It was a mud house. There weren't any pots to cook rice. There was nothing." Her mother managed everything in the beginning, bringing pots and pans, oil, and kerosene. Gradually she returned to her normal chores. When she went to visit her mother for Mother's Day (*aamaako mukh herne din*), she happened to meet a younger friend on the road. Her friend looked at her and said, "Your daughter is small, and yet you have another baby in your stomach or what?" Her friend is a little "over smart." "I said that my menstruation hadn't started yet, and so probably not. And my friend said, 'Really? It can happen before the menstruation starts. How dumb of you! You should go to get tested.'" Maya didn't have any idea of where and how to get a check-up, so she asked her friend to tell her everything. She went to Thapathali, and the doctor informed her she was already five months pregnant. "And I cried all day that day. My daughter was so young, she had only just turned one year old, and I felt so upset, so worried." When it came time to give birth, her mother came and took her daughter, and she checked in to Thapathali hospital. Again she had a difficult birth and needed a blood transfusion. She remained in the hospital for eleven days. She contrasted these two birth experiences with the birth of her son. She experienced no trouble while pregnant with him, and it also wasn't a difficult birth. He was born quickly. At the time of her elder daughter, she had no energy because she didn't eat. At the younger daughter's time, there was much swelling and she couldn't walk. When she gave birth to her third child, her son, it was uncomplicated. Moreover, with the birth of a son, "There was a different kind of happiness at home." She was also pleased. "Having a daughter the first time didn't make any difference; but after having a daughter the second time, I hoped it would be a boy." In fact, her husband had not wanted her to have another child after her second, but she wanted to have one more. And now whenever her son does something wrong, her husband says that they had him because *she* wanted to. "My son is impossible," she said after we laughed. "He gets angry too often. He also doesn't study hard. Daughters study, don't get angry, and don't say, 'I need this, I need that.' They are so well-behaved."

When reflecting on her experience of pregnancy and birth while living in the joint family, Maya said that she did the same amount of work while pregnant as before. She recalled one day that had brought her to tears. She hadn't eaten that morning, for it was the anniversary of a death in the family (*saraadde*). At the morning mealtime she had to go to the field to plant without eating, and Saasu didn't come to take her place until in the evening when it was time to wash the dishes from the evening meal. "I wanted to cry so much. They knew what it was like for me at that time. Only when it was time to wash dishes did BuDhi Saasu go to take my place, and then when I reached the house I wanted to sleep. And at the time I thought I might rest, I was told to go cut fodder. I had to wash dishes, go to cut grass; I had to do everything of course." Remembering another story about her saasu's disregard for her and her eldest daughter's health, Maya described how her parents-in-law wouldn't give her any oil to moisturize the baby's skin. Her daughter's skin was cracked and bleeding, it was so dry, but her parents-in-law said there wasn't even any oil to put on the vegetables (to fry them for meals). And so they refused to give it to her. Ultimately she stole the oil that she was supposed to feed to the young goats they raised and used that for her daughter's skin. In another story about her saasu, Maya told how Saasu had given birth to eleven or twelve children at home. So when Maya needed to go to the hospital, her saasu told her to quit acting (*swaang*). Saasu said, "You're not having an elephant. You're not having a horse. Why are you acting?" But things were changing quickly, for the younger *buhaaris* in the joint household were taken for monthly prenatal check-ups and gave birth in the hospital.

Since a new wife occupies the lowest status in a joint family, women's first pregnancies and births were typically marked with a lack of knowledge and power. Various details in Maya's story demonstrate how she was not able to advocate for her own health or the health of her firstborn daughter. During pregnancy, she was not able to eat due to a combination of not desiring the food items available in the house and not being able to obtain alternatives, having to complete her chores, and being required to follow fasting rules on particular occasions. Hers is a dramatic example, and yet several other women described the cycle of not desiring the delicious but strong-smelling meal eaten twice a day—*daal bhaat*—and vomiting as a result of not eating. Women suffered from the effects of poor nutrition through night blindness, weakness, and dizziness, as well as more nausea. Sita, a mother in her thirties with two girls (HH #135 wife of middle son), described how after the pregnancy nausea started and she did not feel like eating,

> Just like when sick, one's arms and legs feel exhausted, and one wants to keep sleeping. That's what happens. The person will become thin, won't want to eat, feels like spitting, and nausea comes regularly, as

well as dizziness from time to time. I discovered that's how it is. If one becomes weak while pregnant, then the feeling of not wanting to eat will be even stronger. Sometimes after sitting, when I'm about to get up to do some work, [I] feel dizzy and can't see—[I] see black and blue. And because of dizziness I have to sit. After a few moments, after half an hour, it became alright. While being weak it will be like that. In the beginning [of the pregnancy] it was like that.

She also described how her first baby was "born with his stomach stuck to his back," and how the hospital attendants scolded her for not eating enough during pregnancy.

Most women reported eating the same things during pregnancy as they usually did—whatever was available to the household depending on what was in the garden and the amount of money available to purchase things like chicken, goat, or vegetables trucked in from surrounding rural areas. Some older women, as well as Maya, joked about having to eat *DhiDo*, a sticky mass of ground wheat (or corn or millet) with little appeal in terms of taste or texture, because rice was not plentiful year-round and many families could not afford to purchase rice from someone else's fields. DhiDo is joked about as being a poor person's rice. Women reported that they did not eat smaller portions of choice foods like meat or vegetables, but on the whole family members also did not pay special attention to their nutrition. The exception was during the ninth month of pregnancy when traditionally a woman's natal family brings her yogurt, beaten rice, and sometimes fruit and sweets. Several women mentioned that their natal families were unable to fulfill this obligation due to living far away. Overall, not having enough nutritious food for the family as a whole was often the source of women's trouble obtaining adequate nutrition during pregnancy. However, their low status exacerbated such problems because they could not request special foods—meaning something different from what the rest of the family was eating—during periods of nausea.

As for work, many women reported that their household and agricultural duties did not change after they learned they were pregnant. Much like Maya's saasu, one elderly woman (HH #71), the wife of a Gurkha soldier, made light of the whole affair of birth, saying, "If tomorrow I was to give birth, up until today I would be carrying a load of firewood and fodder from that forest (pointing several miles up the mountainside); there, where it is foggy, I would reach that point." I hesitate to call this woman "elderly" since that word carries negative connotations of weakness, and she looked fit and strong. One day she bet that if she wrestled Meena she would win. I agreed. She claimed that it was easy to give birth, and that other than at the time of her first son's birth, she was in labor for only an hour each time.

Boasting about the ease of giving birth and trying to make us laugh, she joked dryly, "I gave birth just like defecating." Regarding the relationship between working and carrying loads and giving birth, she declared, "However much work is done, it becomes that much quicker." According to the mothers-in-law in this study, birth was not something about which to make a fuss. But changes in such beliefs were happening rapidly, sometimes even within a single generation. In Maya's case, the younger women who later married into her husband's ghar were taken for prenatal check-ups and hospital births. These increases in prenatal visits and hospital births were trends evident among the other families in Vishnupura, as well as at the national level, according to the Nepal Demographic and Health Survey (DHS) (Ministry of Health and Population et al. 2007).

Other women who engaged in the same amount of physical labor during pregnancy explained it in terms of necessity. One mother-in-law stated in a matter of fact way, "Who would do the work if I didn't do it?" She had no children old enough to assist her, and her mother-in-law was living with another relative during the time she gave birth. She asked, "How could I get food to eat without doing work? I also had livestock and fields. I had to cut fodder and cook... fetch water... When pregnant, if possible the person will rest; if not—what to do?" Several mothers-in-law followed their explanations of working out of necessity with admonishments that staying active up until the end of pregnancy made the births easier or faster, but overall women's stories about engaging in physically demanding work while pregnant were mixed. Working hard during pregnancy often went hand-in-hand with insufficient nutrition and rest, as well as the inability to get assistance or refuse tasks. Thus even though physical labor may have kept their pregnant bodies strong and healthy in some instances, a woman's low status as a new wife was associated with being overburdened with physically demanding work, often until the end of pregnancy.

Like first pregnancies, first births occurred in a context of limited power and knowledge for young wives in Vishnupura (with the exception of those few who were highly educated), for typically birth occurred at home without the aid of a trained assistant or midwife. This was true at the national level, as well. When considering the socio-historical conditions of the time when the mothers-in-law were giving birth, in the 1980s and 1990s, the reasons for this are clear. Vishnupura was still a rural village at that time and lacked paved roads and electricity. Women had always given birth at home prior to that point, for there were no options or reasons to do it elsewhere. One woman's (HH #106 Saasu) experience of giving birth around 1985 illustrates the context at that time. After being in labor for three days, her father-in-law walked down to call for a vehicle to take her to the hospital. During the time he was gone, she managed to give birth successfully. She explained, "And at that time, just barely, the practice of taking women to the hospital for birth had started. As much as they could, women would give birth at home—but rich people could take the woman to the hospital if the birth was difficult." In her time, taxis were not available. One had to walk to a prestigious boarding school that happened to be located nearby in order to access a phone. Then one could call the hospital to send a vehicle. Another woman (HH #103) found herself in a similar situation a few years later in 1992. She described how when the placenta would not come out, she and her newborn had to be carried on a man's back in a Doko filled with straw down the mountainside until they reached a taxi stand. In addition, I heard the stories of giving birth on the path on the way home from the fields or in the kitchen garden adjacent to the home.[4]

Although these stories of the past struck these women's teenage daughters as strange and foreign, such scenarios would not be uncommon in rural, remote areas of contemporary Nepal. Emergency transport schemes in rural areas of Nepal still utilize bicycle ambulances or Doko (Barker et al. 2007). And the vast majority (81 percent) of births still occurred at home in Nepal during the period of this study when the younger women, the buhaaris, were giving birth. Most women who had given birth in the five years prior to the 2006 DHS reported that they believed it was not necessary to give birth in a health facility (73 percent), 17 percent said it was not customary, 10 percent cited that it cost too much in a health facility, and 9 percent said that a health facility was too far or there was no transportation. In addition, 3 percent of women mentioned that they gave birth before they could get to a facility even though they had planned to for delivery (Ministry of Health and Population et al. 2007). Birth had not been medicalized to the extent that it was viewed as something that had to occur in a health facility even in areas where hospitals and health posts were available.

In rural, remote parts of Nepal health facilities are unavailable, understaffed, or undersupplied. Vishnupura, however, is located on the outskirts of urban Kathmandu, so community members had the option of going to the teaching hospital located nearby, or any of the hospitals located in central Kathmandu or on the southern side, in Patan, if transportation and traffic were both amenable. In sum, available health care facilities for antenatal and delivery care varied in terms of distance and quality. Some women from Vishnupura utilized the teaching hospital, approximately twenty minutes away by public bus and reached much more quickly by taxi, motorcycle, or ambulance. Opinions about the teaching hospital were mixed. Although most complaints were related to long lines, one woman told of a botched stitching by a medical student of a vaginal tear after delivery, which then had to be removed and repeated, and another narrated a close call with another postpartum woman taking her newborn son. A couple of women reported travelling to the maternity hospital in Thapathali, a neighborhood on the southern side of Kathmandu just prior to reaching Patan, and a few went all the way to Patan Hospital. It took anywhere from forty-five minutes to over an hour to reach there from Vishnupura by taxi or car, depending on traffic. Travelling there by bus included at least two changes of vehicles and substantially more time. Thapathali and Patan hospitals had better reputations than the teaching hospital. Closest of all, there was a government sub-health post just downhill from the village, about a fifteen-minute walk from the bazaar, but no one reported going there for antenatal or delivery care. Private hospitals were out of reach economically for the middle- and lower-class families in my research, but wealthy families in or near urban centers like Kathmandu have that option.

Since poverty and/or low status led to problems such as poor nutrition and caloric intake, women were not always positioned positively to give birth at home, unaided. Maya's story of her first birth, which started as a homebirth until there were complications, shared key elements with those of other women in the community. In her case, her parents-in-law were of the opinion that birth did not require a hospital visit. Saasu had given birth successfully to many children at home. However, Maya was in poor health at the outset of labor, and after several days of labor she reports that her husband decided she should not stay at home any longer and took her to the hospital.

The fact that husbands were the decision-makers when it came to determining at what point a normal birth at home transformed into an emergency situation and warranted being taken to the hospital was problematic given that men were not involved in the birth process, and in most cases there was no birth attendant present with the authority to make such a declaration. I argue elsewhere (2010b) that while categorically moving birth out of the home and into the hospital is not advantageous for women's well-being, having a trained birth attendant present—or training husbands—is necessary to ensure that obstetric emergencies are recognized and acted upon in a timely manner (regarding the involvement of husbands, see also Mullany 2006, Mullany et al. 2009). In that article I described several additional stories of women encountering difficulty during homebirths, and how, like in Maya's story, it is the husband or perhaps one of his older brothers who declares it is time to go to the hospital. One of the stories is that of the buhaari of the strong, humorous saasu mentioned above. Anjala (HH #71) was in labor for several days with her first child, but she downplayed her condition. She minimized her role and agency in this situation in order to follow the social script of a good daughter-in-law, avoiding the appearance of being demanding.[5] Eventually her husband's elder brother scolded everyone, saying that she should go to the hospital so that they could remove the baby, and they did. It should be noted that this occurred even in a joint family that was notable for its lack of strong hierarchical relationships and division of labor within the household. Her parents-in-law were remarkably supportive of Anjala during her pregnancy, providing her with yogurt, milk, fruit, and lentils, and assisting her with all of her chores.

Another reason for giving birth at home was that babies do not arrive on schedule or at convenient times. A few women who intended to deliver in a hospital told stories about how they did not leave for the hospital in time, and so they gave birth at home. While this might sound like a straightforward problem of dawdling or not being prepared, in several stories it was linked to waiting for a suitable family member to arrive home in order to escort the woman, and in another to a young Chhettri woman (HH #335) not realizing she was in labor. Any number of significant factors can lie behind the oversimplified statement of "not leaving in time." Another common reason for not making it to the hospital, and for giving birth alone, was when labor started in the middle of the night. Devi's first birth, described in Chapter one, occurred in this manner. Shanta (HH #303), a high-caste woman with some training as a community health volunteer, said that when labor started in the middle of the night with her second pregnancy, she thought, "Why give trouble to others at night. Instead I called out to my mother-in-law just before she was born." Her baby came out "easily," but the placenta did not follow. Eventually she was taken to the teaching hospital after the placenta was manually removed and she had hemorrhaged and lost consciousness. One high-caste mother of five (HH #686), in her forties at the time of research, described how she did not know what to expect when she went into labor with her first child in the middle of the night. She went outside to the garden to walk around and avoid disturbing the others in the house. She gave birth there, outside, in the dark. Another high-caste woman in her forties (#402) relayed in a matter-of-fact way that she had given birth to her first child in the fields on the way home after her labor pains began. While the first woman resented her experience in retrospect and compared herself to a stray dog giving birth in the street, the second woman seemed eager to dismiss any potential pity or negative interpretation of her experience and presented herself as strong and capable.

Maya also addresses several important issues related to reproductive decision-making and contraception. From her account, Maya's first two births sound as if they were life-threatening events. This, combined with the fact that she became pregnant with her second daughter unknowingly prior to the return of her menses, resulted in the couple wondering whether they should avoid having any additional children, despite the social value of sons. Maya's husband inquired about the possibility of her undergoing the permanent sterilization operation while she was in the hospital at the second delivery. The doctor, upon hearing that they had two daughters, discouraged them from opting for a tubal ligation for Maya. And Maya reported that later she felt like she desired another child, and was pleased after having a son. She also said something that was repeated by several other mothers: girls are more apt to be more caring towards the parents, while boys misbehaved and gave their parents trouble. Maya's husband teased her that *she* was the one who wanted another child whenever their son misbehaves. These matters will be explored fully in the next chapter on family planning and the chapter on the attitudes of sons.

Becoming a mother secures one's status in a joint family and establishes one as an important contributing member to the family's future. In fact, most women reported that there was an expectation among family members that they would become pregnant within the first year after marriage. Despite the importance of the contribution of children, the level of hardship faced during pregnancy by many women seemed to be due to more than their low socioeconomic status. Low socioeconomic status compounds a young wife's already low status in the family. Cultivating a stronger direct connection between the value of children and supporting a pregnant woman's health could potentially improve maternal health and birth outcomes, even if in small increments, by leveling some of the gendered status differentials in the home. Ultimately, however, families will be constrained in such efforts by lack of access to nutritious foods and just working conditions.

Becoming a Mother-in-Law

Maya had difficulty imagining what it would be like once she became a mother-in-law and brought a buhaari for her son (who was fourteen at that time). She laughed and said that she would probably have many problems after bringing a daughter-in-law into the household. She figured that since she was not able to make her saasu happy in the past, it might be the same. The buhaari who comes might satisfy her even less than she satisfied her saasu. That's a possibility, isn't it? She had not dared to hope that her son would grow up, bring a buhaari through marriage, and provide her with comfort and happiness. She smiled, and joked that she might be the same as her saasu when she became a saasu. "What will happen, how can we know? As much as possible, I have to think it will not be like that, no?

But tomorrow, anything can happen in the relations of saasu and buhaari. It is impossible to keep good relations. There is little possibility of good relations."

Maya did not think that after she received a buhaari that she would be able to rest and have an easy life. She thought that her current life was easier, and wondered what would happen in the future. Society says that one needs a son and a daughter, but that is just a saying and she does not think like that. However, she already had a son, and she admitted that her thinking might be a result of that fact. "If I had not had a son already, I would have also felt like that maybe." Maya thought that it would be best if her son and buhaari could live together (with her and her husband in a joint family) and keep a good relationship. But if they could not, then they should separate. But it would be best to stay together if they could. She intended to treat her buhaari well.

Near the conclusion of many months of interviews with Maya and the other women in my case studies, I asked them about their hopes for the future, including gaining a daughter-in-law and thereby becoming a mother-in-law. Like most of the women, Maya hoped that after her son married he would continue living with her, effectively turning her nuclear family back into a joint family household. She was ambivalent about how this would turn out, however, pointing to her own highly contentious past relationship with her mother-in-law. With a keen sense of self-awareness, she joked that she might not seem any different to her future daughter-in-law than her mother-in-law had seemed to her.

Maya's improvement in her quality of life was related to the split from her parents-in-law's joint family household and thus a life of agricultural labor. Alternatively, women who had not escaped a life of agricultural labor traced the improvement of their positions to changes in their status within the household over time. They attributed improvements in their quality of life to producing capable children and later becoming a mother-in-law. Like Maya, though, they were of two minds regarding modern daughters-in-law.

Shrimati (HH #165), a Brahmin wife of the eldest son in a large joint family and mother of four, exemplified a woman engaged in demanding agricultural production. Shrimati's husband's family (her ghar) owned the most agricultural land out of all the case study families, and her condition represented one extreme in the range of the degree of physical labor performed by women. Her husband had a high-profile job in Kathmandu that did not pay much, so she, the other daughter-in-law in the household, and her children were responsible for almost all of the work in the fields and for the livestock. However the children were attending school and the younger daughter-in-law was pregnant, so most of the physically demanding work fell on her.

Shrimati had strong opinions about the ways economic developments affected men versus women. When asked about her duties in the household, she responded:

What can be done? There are fields. Even if I had studied, then what? There are lots of fields to look after. We daughters were made to do cultivation work in the fields, and now look at the sons— they are lawyers, businessmen, and so on. And look at the plight of daughters—they are married and sent off to the husbands' houses, so if the husbands give them trouble then what will happen to them. If women studied and became independent they would be able to stand on their feet and not be dependent on their husbands. Now, if the husband mistreats them or beats them they are helpless; they have to stick with such men. What I mean is, we women have been disadvantaged. Now our men own vehicles, motorbikes, and a lot of land. They are influential people in the village. But even though they had all that, they did not educate us girls at all. Why? Because they had so much land, they made us work in the fields; and we are what we are, and look what they have become. Among the three sons of my father . . . (the number of motorcycles, brothers, and brothers' sons gets confusing here, but suffice it to say that her brother and their children own many vehicles, a sign of wealth). And now we women have to survive with such great difficulties… Yes, there is a song, something like, "To a woman, the wealth of the maaita is not of any consequence, neither does she have good times in her husband's house." She has to work very hard in both.

Among women involved in agriculture, their hard work and lack of rest reached almost mythic proportions in their conversations, although they conveyed this by speaking in an understated style with knowing glances as opposed to direct boasting. Shrimati typically peppered her commentaries on Nepali society, the position of women, and her own life experiences with references to fate and the resignation and fortitude with which she faced her lot in life. In her observations that women do not benefit from economic improvements, Shrimati was referring to her own generation of women. When talking about the next generation of women, her daughters or future daughter-in-law, she said that education and economic status would have greater impact.

When asked about how her life would change with the introduction of a daughter-in-law, Shrimati began to joke sarcastically about how a modern buhaari could not possibly bring her any happiness. She explained that she was not educated and barely knew the alphabet, but that her son would need an educated buhaari. Educated women, she stated plainly, do not do agricultural work. According to older women, today's young, educated women are stereotypically lazy when it comes to household duties and chores. Shrimati said about her son,

> [Suppose he] marries an educated buhaari. The buhaari doesn't get a job, and she also doesn't work in the fields, thinking, "Saasu will do everything, this is enough for me . . ." Thinking this, she stays in the room with the door closed in the afternoon resting, also not bringing in any income. And about that which my son earns and brings, she says, "Don't give to your mother. Don't give to your father. I need it." That being the case, my son will change, then. I also have to calculate thinking about that.

Continuing among interruptions of poorly suppressed laughter, Shrimati said, ". . . and she'll say to me, 'Hey, Saasu—bring me some tea.' No, she won't even say 'Saasu.' She'll say, 'Hey, servant, make some tea and bring it here.' Isn't it so?" The vast gap in the education—and in a related way, the worldliness—of the upcoming generation of daughters-in-law threatened the old family hierarchies. This reversal of the typical domination by mothers-in-law of their buhaari was a common subject of joking among married women as they looked ahead and envisioned what their sons' wives would be like. They were doubtful that a buhaari would bring them rest and tranquility, yet they thought that it was good for a son and buhaari to live together with them in a joint family.

Like a Potter's Wheel:
Women and the Patrilocal Cycle

Maya's story helps elucidate the changes in status and identity that occur over time with major transitions in a woman's life—marriage, motherhood, and becoming a mother-in-law—and how they impact her health. Rather than an ahistorical cycle, it becomes clear that changes were occurring in these life course statuses. Maya herself recognized this when reflecting on the differences between her experiences and those of the daughters-in-law who married into the family after her. This begs the question, why do certain gendered truths change in a community while others do not? The following conversation begins to address this question. It captures changes and continuities in gender roles between two generations as they are subtly negotiated by junior and senior female family members in one another's presence. This conversation unfolded one afternoon on the patio of a land-owning Thakuri joint family (HH #77).

Their home was located up the mountainside a ways, and if one peeked over a small plot of corn growing in front of the patio, one had a sweeping view of the Kathmandu Valley below. This household was slightly atypical in a way that was difficult to pinpoint. The members of the household always seemed to be in flux, in their physical presence in the home, whether or not a certain person was mentioned as a member, and how their relation was defined.[6] The core members of the family, who I name according to their kinship status, were the aged but able matriarch (Saasu) and patriarch; their eldest son, his wife (Jethi Buhaari), and their three children; their youngest son, his wife (Kaanchi Buhaari), and their daughter. Only the women and Kaanchi's young daughter were present that day, along with a neighboring mother-in-law (Neighbor Saasu) also of the Thakuri caste and a friend of Saasu. The neighboring saasu was also one of the families I worked with closely (HH #80), but in order to aid comprehension of the conversation I simply refer to her as Neighbor Saasu. This choice of labels is in no way dehumanizing, for people do not use proper names in everyday interactions. I shorten Jethi Buhaari and Kaanchi Buhaari to Jethi and Kaanchi, just as a neighbor might do when referring to the two daughters-in-law. *JeThi* means eldest and *kaanchhi* means youngest, and the "i" on the end of the words signifies that these are women.[7] Kaanchi was officially the one being interviewed when this conversation occurred; otherwise she probably would not have taken the lead in responding (evident in the first portion of the transcript) since she was the lowest in status. She gradually grew quiet, until we returned to the semi-structured format of the interview questions that addressed her directly. I privilege the women's words, tangents, and explanations in the following text, rather than my analysis. Instead of selecting and abstracting quotes relevant to my argument, I prioritize the conversation as it unfolded.

The framing question for the discussion that follows was, "In your opinion, how do women have to be in this society? According to your culture, how do women have to behave?" This question came an hour or two into the interview session, and by this point an air of playfulness had developed, along with sarcasm and teasing that was typical among the women of this particular family. In a similar way to how the women ribbed my research assistant and me, Meena capitalized on the lighthearted mood to press the women of a few of their responses. The discussion was accompanied by raucous laughter, typically absent in individual interviews with women and especially young women. An element of performance was operating in the discussion that afternoon—a performance by the local women for the outsiders, but also for one another's enjoyment (sometimes at the outsiders' expense) and to negotiate their respective positions.

It resulted in a comical portrayal of the difference between the paths of men and women.

JETHI BUHAARI: How do they have to be? For some it will be this way, for some it will be that way.

MEENA: Despite that, in society how does one have to be to be a good person?

KAANCHI BUHAARI: Good…

NEIGHBOR SAASU: Society says to be literate, study, be experienced, get a job, earn money, do housework, mind *saasu* and *sasuraa*, and society will like them. If one is lazy and sits inside one's room all the time, [people] will say [that person is] lazy. (*laughs*)

KAANCHI: Around here we have to work, eh?

NEIGHBOR SAASU: And what to do, then! We have to work. That's how it is!

(*Kaanchi and Neighbor at same time*)

KAANCHI: For doing that they will say, "Good;" and for someone who doesn't do that, "Bad."

NEIGHBOR: Feeding, offering drinks, respecting guests when they come, if everything is done, for that "good" is said. If when there are guests one sits being grumpy, if there is housework and one goes into one's room and sits, what's the use of such laziness?

MEENA: In your opinion, then, if women do all of the housework, society approves.

KAANCHI: Yes.

MEENA: Even if they have studied (been formally educated)?

JETHI: No matter what.

MEENA: And with sons, even if they don't do any work, it will be fine.

KAANCHI: Boys mean boys.

MEENA: Why then?

KAANCHI: Doesn't being a boy or a girl make a difference then?

SAASU: The work boys do will be separate. The work that women do will be separate.

KAANCHI: Women will have housework; boys will have other work.

JETHI: Boys don't get up in the morning and *potne* (cover the floor with a fresh layer of a mixture of mud and cow dung, a traditional job of daughters-in-law first thing in the morning, usually before dawn), it doesn't suit them. (*others laugh*)

MEENA: Why?

JAN: (*laughing*) Why not?

MEENA: Why doesn't it suit them?

JAN: It doesn't suit them?

SAASU: It also doesn't suit them to wash clothes.

JETHI: It doesn't suit them, and what to do?

MEENA: Why doesn't it suit them?

JETHI: Everything suits us, being daughters (women). [Except] we can't go outside and earn income.

MEENA: Why? You all go to *melaa*, work in the fields...[8]

JETHI: That melaa... Then again, we don't know how to hoe. We only plant, and sons (men) continue to hoe. And boys do the work of boys, and girls do the work of girls.

MEENA: Then again, even if boys don't do work for a day, it doesn't make any difference. Being a daughter or buhaari, there won't even be one minute without work.

JETHI: For us it is always the same. Getting up tomorrow morning, that (work); getting up day after tomorrow, exactly that. (*laughs*)

SAASU: Women's housework means...

JETHI: (*looking around for dramatic effect*) Where are the sons who live in this house? Where?

The women subscribe to separate spheres of work and responsibilities between men and women, a clear gender-based division of labor, but they playfully mock it at the same time. The chore described by Jethi of wiping the hard, dry mud floor with a fresh layer of watery mud in the morning, a familiar task to women in days past and in rural areas, seemed so utterly feminine that the image of a man doing such work caused her and the others to laugh. She employs the language "it doesn't suit them" as an explanation, but she notes the limits of that explanation by following it with the joke that everything suits women. She ends by pointing out that there were no men in sight at the house that afternoon. All of them had left for various destinations, not necessarily related to work. In some cases men's absence from the home during the day was due to either agricultural or salaried jobs, but even when they are not working men will not stay at home during the day. They can be found in tea shops, visiting with other men, or younger men often ride into Kathmandu to mill around.

The conversation continued,

SAASU: After having sons and daughters who can do everything, don't we get to sit carefree? If there had been no sons and daughter, [I] would have had to do even that which [I] can't do, dragging myself [I'd] have to do it. I have sons and daughters-in-law, grandchildren, and they will do it.

NEIGHBOR SAASU: For that a son and daughter-in-law is necessary.

SAASU: Yes. For that a son and grandchildren are necessary. A buhaari is needed.

MEENA: That means, women have to do however much work they get, eh?

KAANCHI: Have to.

MEENA: Whether educated or not.

KAANCHI: Despite however much they're educated, they have to clean the baby's shit after having a baby. Who will clean it, then?

MEENA: Husband shouldn't clean as well?

JETHI: He shouldn't.

MEENA: Why?

JETHI: It doesn't suit them. (*with sarcasm—pause while all laugh*) Do boys wear this (sari or skirt)? We wear like this, and it suits us.

MEENA: (*joking*) These days they wear, they wear it.

JETHI: And they don't wear this, boys (*gesturing toward her jewelry*).

JAN: (*joking*) Earrings, necklace—they wear.

JETHI: Boys don't wear saris. How could it suit them! Boy and girl were sent differently from up above. And don't we have to distinguish?

JAN: How did it become that way?

JETHI: Who knows!

KAANCHI: How, how!

JETHI: How, how. I don't know. From ancient times the traditions have been like this. Who knows, no?

MEENA: But compared to before it has become a little different, probably.

JETHI: Now it has a little, by educating, listening.

SAASU: Before, people…

JETHI: Now there are educated people who say boys and girls should work equally, no? Boys and girls work equally, eat equally, wherever they go they walk around equally; in some places that is also true. In village households like ours, it's not like that. In such a village there will be village households. As for in the city, the bazaar, outside— boys and girls walk together. Both wear pants. Boys and girls, no? Here, if our husbands wear pants, do we wear pants? Our [situation] is like that.

MEENA: But long ago people used to always wear a sari (even at home). Now people also wear only this much (*referring to her more informal* lungi *skirt and* cholo *blouse*), isn't it so?

JETHI: Yes.

MEENA: Change occurred.

JETHI: While working in the house we wear [clothing] like this, if we have to go here and there (outside of the village), we wear sari. We carry our bag, and making ourselves look tip top we walk about. Here while doing work with livestock, going to cut fodder, why would we wear sari? We have to work.

MEENA: Yes. Long ago, after getting married you had to cover your head with your sari, no?

JETHI: Yes.

MEENA: And that has changed now, no?

JETHI: Yes. We've already become old, we know everyone, so there is no embarrassment. Long ago one had to cover, I've heard, and . . . (unclear) not show one's head to husband's elder brothers. It was like that. We don't have any husband's elder brothers in our home, then why should we cover the breast that has already been sucked by the baby . . .

A large part of the rationale for having children was the need for a son and daughter-in-law to take over productive tasks once one becomes too aged to do it oneself. Thus the workings of the domestic cycle, the gift of daughters to other families and the receipt of daughters-in-law into the family, and the need for sons in order for this to happen, were explicitly talked about in agricultural families like this one. Although Jethi acknowledged the changes in gender roles in cities, she distinguished rural areas like Vishnupura as being a different case, particularly in terms of dress. She identified equity between the sexes as an urban phenomenon. Similarly, she thinks the education of a woman would not mitigate family duties and chores in a household such as hers.

Later in the interview, she continued with the theme of a sari both representing and hindering women:

For them (men), children don't follow after them. No one gives trouble to men; after saying, "Let's go," they slip on their pants and go. (*Laughs*) After putting on sari, children grab on, immediately, saying, "I will come too!" And where to carry them? Should I carry them on this side, on that side, or walk by myself? (*Mimicking shifting a small child from one hip to the other in an exaggerated fashion, as well as the small steps one has to take while wearing sari.*) What can I do? (*All laugh*) That being the case, I stay at home. Even though I want to go, I stay quietly.

Her saasu supported her, saying, "After mothers say they are going somewhere, the children will also say, 'I want to go!' of course. And in a line

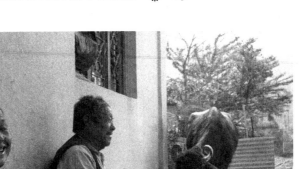

Fig. 6. A mother-in-law of a large multi-generational family smiles as we discuss gender roles.

[they follow after her] . . ." Jethi complained that children cannot walk long distances and that she cannot carry them. Thus she prefers not attempting to go out. Men, on the other hand, "Eat, wash up, and go." Mobility was thus another major distinction between men and women.[9]

The focus of the conversation then shifted to my situation, at that time as a young, unmarried woman. Jethi teased me by saying that I should have two children and then do family planning. This was a brilliant sarcastic application of the family planning message promoted by the government and international non-governmental organizations alike, that "a small family is a happy family," and one should have two children and then "do family planning." Instead of INGOs funded and run by predominantly white Americans or Europeans telling Nepali women how to manage their sex lives and procreation, a Nepali woman with only an elementary-school level of education turned the power structure upside down by teasing a young, white American that she should have two children and then do family planning. It was one of the highlights of my decade of research in this community. This subject will be picked up again in the following chapter.

They teased Meena, as well, for at that time Meena was past what was considered to be a marriageable age and was unmarried. Meena, who has a Master's Degree in Anthropology, was living at home and caring for her aging mother and their household when she was not working as a research assistant or consultant. The women teased Meena that she did not have to work hard because she was unmarried and living at home (though I knew how hard she worked!):

JETHI: (*to Meena*). . . Now because you are still at your maaita you are carefree, you are able to go and travel around, no? After returning home, (your) mother and father say, "Daughter, come here to eat." With ease, no? If we travelled around all day and returned, (Saasu would say) "Here's your rice" (*using "ta" form, a highly disrespectful or "low" verb form*). (*laughs*)

MEENA: Your saasu is laughing!
   (*all laugh*)

JETHI: It is also not her (Saasu's) own home. She left her maaita and came [here], no? Saasu is like that, buhaari is also like that.

KAANCHI: [That's how] it operates/continues/works (*chalchha*).

SAASU: [That's how] it operates/continues/works.

NEIGHBOR SAASU: It's like a potter's wheel. It goes around and around.

JETHI: She also left her maaita and came here. She was not born here. We were also not born here. Leaving one's maaita, one comes. You, also, as long as you stay at your maaita, you are so worry-free, no?

In the discussion of gender in this chapter, we now arrive back at the opening topic of women's positions as daughters in their natal homes. The ease of living in one's maaita is contrasted with life in one's husband's home, but Jethi makes the astute point that the home/household (ghar) in which she lives is also not really her saasu's home. Thus Jethi momentarily levels the typical hierarchical relationship between mother-in-law and daughter-in-law by uniting them under the broader, shared category of being a woman in a patrilocal society—of being a woman who is an outsider in her own home. The circulation of women into and out of a household at the time of marriage and the transition of women through familial and domestic roles are all "like a potter's wheel."

Conclusion

In this research, out of a variety of potential factors that influence women's positions and procreation, the patrilineal, patrilocal features of Hindu-caste Nepali society emerged as some of the strongest and most resistant to change. They buttressed existing gender norms and perpetuated son preference, despite dramatic changes in the education of women and the abandonment of agriculture for other means of production. With each generation in a household, women circulated out of their natal homes and into the homes of their husbands. From the perspective of a household, or that of men (since men constitute the household and do not circulate), this pattern takes on a cyclical appearance. Cyclical not in terms of a life cycle of the type described in biology, but rather as a process that occurs repeatedly over time. While following a single life course trajectory like Maya's, this pattern may not be apparent; but women explained to me again and again that this loss of daughters and gain of daughters-in-law underlay all aspects of family life, including their reproductive desires. And, as an aside, even women in nuclear families almost unanimously voiced a desire for their family to become a joint family again with the marriage of a son.

Despite its fundamentality to social and familial life, the trope of a cyclical potter's wheel belies women's own observations of historical change as well as their ability to resist gender norms. First of all, many of the women did not imagine that they would be better off once they reached the status of mother-in-law, for nowadays daughters-in-law are more educated than they are. This difference in education and worldliness undermined the high status of contemporary mothers-in-law. Thus while this research supports prior conclusions regarding the embodied experience of low status for young wives, it disputes some of the narratives in South Asian scholarship and demography about the dominance of mothers-in-law. Second, a further example arose in the conversation between the members of a joint family and their neighbor. The women mocked the fundamental gender differences to which they subscribe, and for a moment they unified women across various life stages through recognizing their similar plight in contrast to men. All the women of a multi-generational family are technically outsiders, with the exception of the young, unmarried daughters. Despite the hierarchy of power and status among women in a household, they share the quality of being brought into that household through marriage. Even while women emphasized the fundamental role of patrilocality and its enduring nature, they also contradicted that characterization by noting changes over time and their own capacity for disrupting it as a norm. In these ways the potter's wheel trope is useful precisely because although it described a dominant shared understanding of the female gender and patrilocality, its limitations are apparent and were exposed by women as they talked. In order to disrupt a timeless notion of gender roles further, in the next chapter I focus on the specific historical processes that have impacted women's lives.

3

The Elusive Small, Happy Family

While conducting an interview in the warm afternoon sun on a rooftop patio of a three-story concrete building, home to several separate families renting flats, a neighbor interrupted the conversation with her own remarkable story. She boasted that many years ago she had gone to have a tubal ligation (permanent female sterilization operation) after having only two children. A silver-haired woman sitting at a little distance from us on the roof, older than the interviewee and the storyteller, expressed her disbelief. "It's true, I did," the neighbor continued, ". . . and that day after I got the operation, I was lying there saying 'oooh' (from the pain), and at the same time my mother-in-law was saying, '*Mares*' (may you die)." She mimicked for humorous effect the chopping gesture her mother-in-law had made, and the women on the roof all laughed. Her father-in-law had called her sinful, and even her doctor had not approved at first. When she had arrived for the operation, the doctor asked about her children. When he found out she had only two children, both under five years of age, and only one son, he advised her not to have the operation because there was no certainty that the children would survive. After he refused, she said she pleaded, ". . . if they die, may it be so; it doesn't make a difference to me. Do it, do it for me." She claimed that in this way, through her boldness and perseverance, she convinced the doctor to do the operation.

In contrast to the trope of the potter's wheel invoked by the women in the previous chapter, this story underscores the necessity of a historical perspective. At the point in Nepal's history when the neighbor was in her reproductive years, she was clearly expected to have more than two children, and more than one son. She was telling a story of roughly fifteen years prior, around 1989, when Nepal's total fertility rate was 4.79 (Ministry of Health and Population et al. 2002) and infant and child mortality were familiar events. The purpose of this chapter is to unpack the various dominant discourses and structures that led to the shared understanding with which these women tacitly understood that this story was exceptional, knew it was worth telling, and found it amusing.

What may appear to be "local" stories told in this chapter are framed by a critical analysis of the global discourses—in the academy and the international development community—on women, development, and family planning and their evolution over time. In the contemporary state of globality, analyzing such discourses is a necessary step in understanding how women negotiate competing discourses. How international or bilateral organizations such as International Planned Parenthood Federation, USAID, and the United Nations construct the category of women impacts women's most intimate actions. I examine how discourses on family planning impinge upon Nepali women's lives, arguing for an approach to understanding reproductive behavior that allows for the unfolding and improvisational process of reflection and figuring out one's position through speech, action, and inaction.

Global Discourses on Women and Procreation

Women in the global South have been defined and thereby objectified in various ways over the past few decades according to the overriding theoretical assumptions and dominant political players of the time. While, thanks to many feminist and critical theorists, the aspects of a person's position that cross-cut a supposed group such as "women" seems obvious by those of us situated in the early twenty-first century, a brief foray into the ways "Third World" women have been constructed and defined by demographers and development planners is useful in understanding the globalization of historically contingent, Western ideas about population growth and the technologies and initiatives that followed. I do not aim to pass judgment on any individual demographers and development agencies, but to trace the ways in which the global North's concern with human population growth developed and became reconstituted in terms of a concern for reproductive health and women's rights. By foregrounding this history, it then becomes easier to question the particular framing of Nepali women in such terms.

Demography Defines Women

In the realm of population and development planners, women were first equated with fertility itself: as something that needed to be controlled.

During the 1950s and 1960s, reviving Malthusian logic and explaining scarce global resources and poverty in terms of an unchecked human population "explosion" (Ehrlich 1968), intellectuals and political leaders in the United States (U.S.) began to develop programs aimed at reducing what were considered to be high fertility rates in the global South. Historian Tom Robertson (2012) describes how the two key organizations in global efforts at fertility reduction, the Population Council and International Planned Parenthood Federation, were created by individuals who had a mixture of motivations and concerns: global overpopulation and its impacts on the political security and natural resources of the U.S., women's right to contraception, and also some lingering eugenic motivations towards societies and segments of society deemed inferior. To varying degrees, the neo-Malthusians ignored the overconsumption occurring in the global North and the unequal distribution of the world's resources as drivers of the hunger and suffering evident in the world's poorest nations (compare with Hartmann 1995). Nevertheless, the early family planning movement gained momentum and demography became a nascent field of inquiry.

During the 1950s, the Population Council devoted most of its budget to demographic research and training hundreds of officials from countries around the world, which effectively became a global network of American-trained demographers. Historian John Sharpless writes, "the American vision of population studies became the global vision" (1997, 183). Demographers have often tried to distance themselves from the population control movement (see Mason 1995), the political agenda of limiting births in the global South, and some of the blemishes including eugenic measures and questionable testing of contraceptives on populations in the global South. Yet much of their funding came from governments and international agencies that had such agendas (Greenhalgh 1996). Indeed, demography (synonymous with population studies) as an intellectual pursuit and discipline was born out of neo-Malthusian concern about global overpopulation.

In the 1980s and 1990s, women in what were labeled developing countries, a label which betrayed the underlying biased view that industrialized nations were superior and developed and other countries were simply behind on the linear path of so-called progress (see Escobar 1995), began to be portrayed by demographers and development economists as more than fertile objects that needed to be controlled. It was decided that women were rational, thinking, feeling beings who were influenced by testable environmental factors. This represented a significant break from viewing women synonymously with fertility. Women were no less the objects of biopower, in Foucauldian terms (Foucault 1978), of both the state and international population and development agencies, but they gained an increase in the recognition of their human dignity and agency. For example, sterilization campaigns and unethical experimental trials in the global South were no longer acceptable, but the control of populations and fertility remained the underlying objective: the hegemonic aspiration of lowering fertility continued to drive much population policy and funding.[1] Scholars turned their focus to defining the concepts of women's status and autonomy, and testing the relationship of variables such as education, control over resources, and employment outside of the home in a search for the salient variables that lead to higher status. They found that social and institutional denial of women's equal access to and control over resources were associated with high rates of fertility worldwide. The improved status of women was hypothesized to result from increased educational or economic opportunities (Caldwell 1982), both leading to fertility decline. These models were rather homogenous and unidirectional in their explanations, however, and were challenged in this regard. Karen Mason (1986, 1987) was a forerunner in pointing out the failure of social demographers to recognize the multidimensionality of women's status and its variation across social locations, for example differences in status in the household versus in the community, or across the various stages of the life course.

Change in women's status can be multidirectional, as well, improving in some realms and worsening in others, as traditional norms and behaviors that protected women break down (Bradley 1995). In regard to relative life expectancies between men and women, Amartya Sen pointed out (1990) that economic development is often accompanied by a relative worsening in the survival rates of women. In India women's relative positions deteriorated with the onset of economic development for decades until the gap between the life expectancy of men and women narrowed within the last few decades (Sen 1990). In such cases, women may not have access to or benefit from advances in health services and infrastructure and general economic progress. New practices can also reinforce established attitudes towards gender roles rather than changing them. Ahearn's ethnographic research in a Magar village in Nepal illustrates how increased female literacy rates, for example, do not automatically lead to better lives for women (Ahearn 2001). While education may be related to a decrease in fertility, it is not necessarily related to an increase in power for women. Mainstream demography rarely took note of such microlevel analyses of reproduction, however, despite their capacity to complicate and enhance the understanding of so-called fertility behavior (Kertzer and Fricke 1997; Connelly 2003).

The growing concern for the status of women across the globe was evidenced within the development world by the 1994 International Conference on Population and Development (ICPD) by the "empowerment of women" becoming the catchphrase of the conference and by the presence of a

large contingency of organizations involved in women's rights. The resulting ICPD Program of Action recognized reproductive health and rights,
and women's empowerment more broadly, as cornerstones of a successful population and development program. The following year in Beijing,
the Fourth World Conference on Women, as its name implies, focused
more broadly on women's rights. The platforms established at Cairo and
Beijing "converge in their affirmation of women's human rights and the
recognition that solving the world's most pressing problems demands
the full participation and empowerment of the world's women" (United
Nations Population Fund). The shift in the discourse from an explicit
neo-Malthusian agenda to one that espoused women's rights and well-
being solidified around this time.

Despite some progress in the way social scientists were defining wom-
en's status, it remained a limited concept because it concentrated too heavily on structure and was not well suited to account for women's agency or
the contingent and fluid nature of social processes. Moreover, a multitude
of voices called for the disposal of any such universal category because
of the inherent flaws.[2] Third World Feminists and Subaltern theorists
denounced and deconstructed such universal and homogenizing categories as "women," based on their inadequacy to capture diversity in women's
experiences and the complex ways women experienced oppression based
on multiple aspects of their identity.[3] In her comprehensive review of what
feminist contributions could offer to the field of demography, Riley concluded that evidence and research called for "culturally grounded research
on gender that does not assume that Western notions of any institutions or
concepts, including gender, status, and power, are necessarily similarly valued or interpreted in societies" (1999, 382–383). I turn now from the project
of tracing the act of defining "women" from the perspective of social scientists and policy planners concerned with development and fertility decline,
to the example of how these dominant ideas and policies circulating in the
global North impacted Nepal.

Demography's Story of Fertility Decline in Nepal

In countries around the world, demographers observed that fertility transitions have been associated with economic growth and social change.
According to John Caldwell, a demographer well-known for his theories
of fertility decline, the onset of fertility transition has followed "the conversion of economies into ones where practically all transactions are mon-
etized, where children go to school, where modern medical facilities are
easily available, where an increasing number of mothers received trained
health professional assistance when giving birth, and where infant and

child mortality rates are falling to at least moderate levels" (1998). In such a context, children become expensive and the allocation of resources within a family shifts (Caldwell 1982). This ideology itself—the whole-hearted adoption of it and the translation of it into funded programs by international organizations and Nepali policy-makers—may have influenced fertility decline in Nepal as much as the actual conditions described by it.

A demographic story of fertility decline in Nepal goes something like this. Nepal is a nation of disparities, and this is reflected in fertility differentials. There is a small educated, wealthy, and worldly elite class on one end of the spectrum, and a rural and impoverished majority on the other end. The lives of these two extremes are utterly different, and the study population addressed in this research represents the middle ground. Many of the cities in the middle hills and the Tarai (the southern plains) regions are becoming part of a global economy and society, and Kathmandu almost fully so. The mountainous region that stretches the northern length of the country offers a formidable challenge to the development of infrastructure and the provision of services like education and health care, or even roads. Consequently, fertility rates are lower in urban areas, which are concentrated in the middle hills and Tarai, among the well educated, and among the wealthy.

Despite the country's status as one of the world's poorest and the challenges of its extreme topography to development, Nepal has undergone a fertility transition. The total fertility rate declined from over 6 births per woman of reproductive age in the 1970s, to 3.1 in 2006 (Ministry of Health and Population et al. 2007).[4] This drop in fertility occurred despite high infant mortality rates and problems with both access and quality of care for women during delivery. According to the 2006 Demographic and Health Survey, the infant mortality rate and the under-five mortality rate, though dropping, were high at 48 and 61 (per 1000 live births) respectively. Acute respiratory infections and diarrheal diseases were the most prominent killers of infants. The large majority of women (81 percent) gave birth at home between the 2001 and 2006 DHS, many without the assistance of a trained professional.

Contributing to fertility decline was the marked increase in the use of temporary methods of contraception between 1996 and 2006. Historically sterilization had accounted for the largest share of contraceptive use in Nepal, but initially this may have been attributable to the emphasis placed on this method by family planning programs and subsequently local practitioners or field workers (see Appendix B: Trends in Contraceptive Use in Nepal). Although it was popular, permanent contraception was used (primarily by women) with caution, as the experience of child death was not uncommon. The age at marriage also increased, another condition for fertility decline, but the median age at first birth had changed very little in the past two decades—remaining at 20 years of age (Ministry of Health and Population et al. 2007).

The pace of economic development has been slow for Nepal, and was impeded further by political events, civil unrest, and the intensification of the Maoist People's War between 2001 and 2006. The violence and fear caused by the insurgency and the army's response also increased the divide between life in urban and remote rural areas. Most of the fighting took place in the rural countryside, and a substantial number of men fled to urban areas and sometimes abroad in order to escape the violence and find employment. The drop in fertility documented by the 2006 DHS may be driven, at least in part, by the resulting separation of couples or the movement of couples from rural to urban areas.

With opportunities for education, employment, and new forms of leisure, the costs and benefits of childrearing change and individuals are exposed to new ideas that may influence fertility behavior in Nepal (Axinn 1992; Axinn and Yabiku 2001), as well as across many societies (Thornton and Fricke 1987). In semi-urban areas like the one described here, the transition away from agricultural labor as the main means of production towards small businesses or various wage-paying positions was well underway. People recognized the value of education, plus the costs associated with it, although they often expressed discouragement over education not resulting in employment.

In summary, the total fertility rate for women of reproductive age in Nepal fell from around six children per woman to three within two generations. The major causes of this fertility decline, according to a demographic perspective, are the promotion, availability, and acceptability of contraception and related services, along with the structural conditions described above. The question of *why* lower fertility and the utilization of contraception became acceptable remains. Meta-narratives such as the demographic transition theory miss individuals' lived experience and potential to act in creative ways, reducing fertility to structural influences. Fertility transition theories cannot account for why certain beliefs and traditions that relate to fertility are abandoned while others are not. For these reasons, I will describe some of the specific historical developments along with women's own stories of negotiating various discourses on how they ought to produce.

The "Small, Happy Family" in Nepal

Historically, the acceptability of limiting family size was driven by a dramatic expansion of the role of the state into everyday affairs, in particular into

Nepalis' reproductive lives. This began in 1959 with the establishment of the first family planning service organization, the Family Planning Association of Nepal (FPAN). The following year FPAN became an associate member of International Planned Parenthood Federation. Around the same time, the government of Nepal began to associate the role of family planning with national development and family welfare. The government concluded that reducing the national fertility rate would help maintain a balance between population growth and economic growth, and so it adopted a family planning policy in 1965. Subsequent development plans dealt with population processes from both a policy and programmatic point of view. From 1985 to 1990, population policies and programs not only emphasized family planning issues in the short term, but also focused on long-term concerns such as encouraging the small family norm through education and employment programs that aimed to raise women's status and decrease infant mortality. The government altered its position from encouraging family planning through sterilization to promoting temporary methods. The Eighth Plan (1992–1997) continued the strategy to create a favorable atmosphere for the small family norm of two children through economic and development programs and improve the scope and quality of family planning services offered throughout the country, but it also established a new emphasis on the concept of birth spacing and the use of temporary birth control methods (Government of Nepal 1992, 350). The Ninth Plan (1997–2002) promoted the slogan "Small Family for Happy Family" to the rural populace and aimed to reduce population growth through improvement in the health of women and children (Government of Nepal 1997, 635).

Governmental and private organizations' pro- family planning and small family position is evident in the media and even in the school curriculum. Tatsuro Fujikura describes (2004) how large billboards began to appear in Kathmandu's urban landscape in the late 1990s, including ones for Sangini, the local brand of hormonal contraceptive injection that lasted three months. He cites a USAID report describing its Contraceptive Retail Sales project that began in the late 1970s as including innovative contests and displays, such as a Frisbee contest held in the national stadium and a float in King Birendra's birthday parade. Such programs aimed to increase public awareness of contraceptives and reduce social resistance to the subject (Skerry et al. 1991, cited in Fujikura 2004). And in the remote, rural village of western Nepal where he conducted research in the late 1990s, Fujikura was struck by the ubiquity of the presence of family planning messages on posters, in print and radio advertisements, and even in conversations among villagers. Development discourses, in this instance those regarding small families and contraceptive use, shape people's sense of self as well as their relations to others (cf. Kunreuther 2006; Pigg 1992).

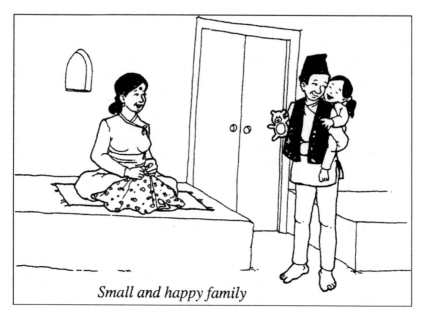

Small and happy family

Fig. 7. Depiction of the small and happy family. From the textbook *Our Environment and Population*, for Class 6. The caption reads, "With the help of family planning measures, a man can get the desired number of children. It helps a small family. The small family is a happy family. The mother and child are safe in a small family. It is difficult to fulfill the wants if there are many sons and daughters in the family. Thus, the family suffers."

During the span of my research, advertisements for family planning were found throughout the Kathmandu Valley on buses, taxis, and billboards, and on the radio, on television, and in newspapers. As early as grade five, school children began to learn the importance of family planning for the development of the country, and the difference between permanent and temporary methods of contraception. By grade six, children learned more about various methods of contraception as well as the reasons why a small family is a happy family (Figure 7).

In the textbook "Our Environment and Population" for class seven, an illustration depicts a family planning camp bearing the slogan, "small family, happy family" (Figure 8). Mobile sterilization camps, including an operating tent and all the necessary medical supplies, moved throughout rural areas, offering sterilization operations for women and men. Sterilization was the means of contraception preferred by governmental and private organizations in remote areas where there were inadequate medical services to offer a choice of temporary methods of family planning. The text accompanying the image of the family planning camp reads, "The family planning is one of the important measures to control the growth of

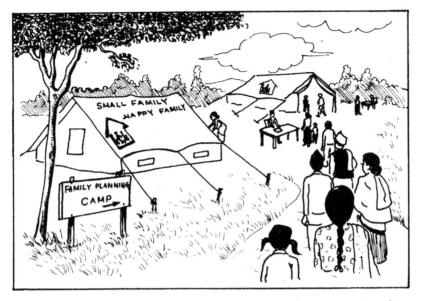

Fig. 8. Depiction of the small family, happy family slogan at a sterilization camp. From the textbook, *Our Environment and Population*, for Class 7.

population. It helps to make a small and happy family. It helps people to produce a limited number of children in the right time. The need of education, health, food, clothing, etc. can be made available if the number of children is small. If the number of children is large, it will be difficult to fulfill every need of the children and their life will be miserable." The same textbook for class eight discusses the "culture of low fertility": how "industrially advanced countries," the rich countries of Europe, North America, and Japan, prefer small families. "They are happy and satisfied with one or two children. 'A new baby or a new car' is their motto. So often they decide in favour of the car." Above and beyond encounters with family planning messages through school and advertising, the general exposure to new ideas through an increase in the prevalence of education, through encounters with global media (see Liechty 2003), and through a general trend in the consumption of modernity in the terms of development created a favorable context for the acceptability of modern methods of contraception.

The women in the case study families were familiar with the "happy family," two-child model that was commonly promoted on radio and television, and referenced the slogan in our conversations. Since their establishment in Nepal in the 1960s, internationally funded family planning organizations as well as the Ministry of Health spread the message that a small family was a happy family, a slogan that can be heard in different languages throughout the developing world. And indeed, women talked about

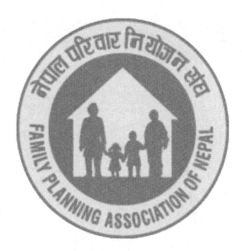

Fig. 9. The logo of the Family Planning
Association of Nepal, depicting a
family with one son and one daughter.

two, otherwise three, children being enough. Yet there is a problem with
the "happy family" representation, a serious inherent contradiction that is
apparent in the very logo of the Family Planning Association of Nepal: the
image of two parents with two children, one daughter and one son. The
presence of one son was crucial in this context. How can a family ensure
such a perfect composition of offspring as in the logo (Figure 9)? Only
roughly 50 percent of couples would produce the sex composition of the
children in the FPAN logo, one girl and one boy. Another 25 percent would
produce two boys, and the remaining 25 percent would produce two girls.
The logo therefore encapsulates the way many contemporary young mothers were faced with conflicting discourses: produce a son, but only have
two children. Notably, India attempted to avoid this problem in some of its
family planning images, releasing a two rupee coin with the small family,
happy family logo in 1993 that strategically depicted two female children,
as well as postage stamps in 1994, one of which depicted only one female
child. FPAN had released a similar stamp in 1984, featured on the cover of
this book; but it featured one boy and one girl.

"Son Preference"

Women debated the need for sons; some debated internally, some debated
it with other women in their household in my presence, and some thought
that there was no debate—of course a family needs to produce sons. Some
women proclaimed defiantly, "What good are sons?!" but most conceded
that they *were* good. More accurately, they were necessary. And young
women who had sons were relieved to be exempt from the discussion
having any implications for them.

In demography, the concept of son preference was developed to describe a phenomenon that demographers observed in patriarchal societies all over the world, in which families preferred and celebrated the birth of sons over daughters. According to the mothers in this study, the term son preference mischaracterizes the situation. Women do not prefer sons to daughters; rather they feel compelled to produce a son. In the context of dramatically lower fertility in comparison with the previous generation, however, the pressure to produce a son had become more acute as young women felt it necessary to give birth to a male in fewer overall attempts. This condition is referred to in the title of the chapter, the elusive "small, happy family." Women find themselves in the middle of these disparate discourses, and through their procreation they enact both social continuity and change.

The Rhetoric of Mothers-in-Law about Sons

According to the older generation of women (the mothers-in-law), sons were necessary for a family for two reasons: for performing funeral rites and bringing a daughter-in-law into the family. In discussions of the necessary number of children one should have, the presence or absence of sons in the formula always changed the end sum. Many women said about their daughters-in-law, "This generation gives birth to up to three, no? Why have more than that?" When asked what if all three children were daughters, the common reply was, "If they are all daughters? One son is needed. One son is needed for the funeral rites." Most members of this older generation agreed that a son was needed during the funeral rites to light his parents' pyres and ensure their passage from this world to the next. This is an important and pervasive Hindu belief, yet people had difficulty explaining the significance behind the tradition and why it mattered. One Brahmin woman (HH #402), the wife of a respected local Hindu priest, was one of the only individuals who knew, or had seriously considered, the reasons behind the tradition:

> We need one son because without a son we cannot do anything when the parents die. A daughter cannot perform her parents' funeral rites according to our religion. A son has to perform them . . . Whatever no-good drunkard, thief, and gambler a son may be, society cannot have funeral rites without a son. Even at the time of death you need a son, because daughters are married off to other houses; they will not be able to come home at the time of an emergency. From that point of view, too, a son is badly needed. Otherwise there won't be a single person to give you a drop of water on your deathbed. Who will take care of the parents in the family if a son is not there?

Mothers-in-law claimed that if families were lacking a son, they had to find a nephew to perform the funeral rights; a daughter would not do. However, as with most traditions, situations frequently arise that are far from ideal, a situation in which there is neither son nor nephew, for example. Anecdotally, I heard of brothers and even daughters who lit the pyre.

The other reason that sons are needed, according to mothers-in-law, is because a family's own daughters are lost to other families through marriage, and a son will bring a daughter-in-law into the household. In the lively discussion of gender roles featured in Chapter two, the mother-in-law from the neighboring house (HH #80) summed up the role of daughters. She joked loudly to the group, "The daughter runs off—if she is given away (in an arranged marriage), she goes; if she isn't given away, she goes. If there is a son, he will care [for the parents]." She was making the point that whether a woman elopes or her marriage is arranged, eventually she "runs off" (*bhaagchha*), leaving her parents' household. Everyone recognized the truth of that statement. Sons, on the other hand, remain with their families and care for their parents as they age. Jethi (first introduced in Chapter two, HH #77) added: "After one becomes old, parents, we old people, won't be able to work. [We] can't do fieldwork, can't care for livestock. For that a son is needed. After a son is born, a daughter-in-law will come. After the *buhaari* (daughter-in-law) comes, they will manage things and do the fieldwork. They will have babies. And for these things, isn't a family necessary? Without a son, where does a buhaari come from?"

Sons, therefore, are needed for a much more practical and pressing reason than conducting funeral rites. A son brings a daughter-in-law into the household. More than an issue of religious tradition, the introduction of a daughter-in-law is a matter of acquiring help with daily responsibilities and the functioning of the household and family. The introduction of a daughter-in-law significantly changes the allocation of responsibilities in the household: the matriarch and daughters in the family pass on to the new wife duties such as fetching firewood and fodder, cooking, washing clothes, and cleaning. As described in Chapter two, the new wife bears the greatest burden of time- and labor-intensive domestic duties and suffers the lowest status in the hierarchy of her new family (Bennett 1982; Cameron 1998; Jeffery et al. 1988). Over time, her position improves with the birth of children, especially sons, and the introduction of another young wife into the family by her husband's brother or, eventually, by her own son (cf. Das Gupta 1995).

The following account about her eldest son's wife who left the family out of shame, told by the aged but active mother-in-law (HH #77) featured in the extended conversation in Chapter two, highlights potential dangers to having few or no sons given the current structure of society and demographic realities. One of her daughters-in-law, Kaanchi, began by saying, "During our time, we didn't know about this 'happy family' (*sukhi pariwaar*)." Saasu continued:

> Before [people] didn't know, but now after having two or three children they do family [planning]; although this doing family planning, it doesn't suit some people. It suits some, it doesn't suit others. Our eldest daughter-in-law—her one daughter is still living—she had two sons and then did family planning. The two sons died. And the mother became naked, no? It's like that, it doesn't suit some . . . Her daughter left, and her sons died. And didn't the mother become empty?! It's like that. Now, I don't allow the daughters-in-law to do family planning. However many children they have, they will have. . . . After having them, may they raise them; after they get older, may they earn and eat.

As this story attests, a woman may be left metaphorically "naked," or exposed and vulnerable, and "empty" in society if she produces no sons or loses the ones that were supposed to care for her, according to the older generation of mothers-in-law.

Young Mothers Negotiate Conflicting Discourses

Women who were still reproductively active (meaning those who had not become grandmothers) objected to what "society" said regarding the need for sons. These younger women declared that they did not understand such "traditions" as the requirement that a son must light the funeral pyre. Sita, a young, high-caste mother with two daughters (HH #135 wife of middle son, introduced more fully below), expressed her frustration about feeling pressure to produce a son:

> So, here's my problem. People have no sense. They say that [a son] is needed at the time of death. They say that, "the door will be closed," and so, "the door has to be opened." I can't understand people's talk! "The door will be closed at the time of death if we have only daughters," they say. And if there is a son, whatever kind of son, the door can be opened, it is said. What a thought, such thinking by society! Even if I quit thinking bad things, others will talk badly. Even if one tries to be satisfied oneself, others say bad things. What can you do? Society is like that.

Young wives such as Sita who no longer believed in the unassailability of traditions nevertheless expressed the importance of conforming in order to avoid the scorn and gossip of others.

Most young mothers in Vishnupura downplayed the necessity of having sons, stating that girls were just as good as boys and that they did not favor one over the other. In fact, like Maya in Chapter two, two other women commented that girls were better because of the support that a daughter offers to her mother. One woman said that having a daughter is like having a friend in the home, and another commented that daughters are more attentive than sons. Women who had sons were clearly in a position of being able to deny with ease the importance of sons, whereas the experience of women who did not have a son was entirely different. All of the young mothers in my case studies who did not yet have sons were concerned about whether to give birth again. These young mothers without sons were the ones who had to negotiate the pressure to produce a son.

The pressure on individual women to give birth to sons came from many sources. The value of sons was reinforced subtly through the popular media, such as television serials, and in less subtle ways, for example, by doctors who discourage women from being sterilized if they have only one son, according to the neighbor's story above. Women in Vishnupura experienced the pressure to produce sons most directly through their in-laws, their husbands, sometimes their neighbors, and, notably, through their own self admonitions.

Durga (HH #241), a young, high-caste woman with two daughters, lived in a sizable cement house with her many joint family members. Despite her parents-in-law's strictness, particularly that of her mother-in-law, Durga said that she was the person most disappointed when she gave birth to her second daughter. Although some husbands beat their wives if they do not produce sons, she reported, her husband had said nothing negative to her. She explained: "In fact, when I used to get angry about the daughters, about not being able to have a son, their daddy used to convince me that there is no difference between son and daughter. The second time when I gave birth to a daughter, he told me not to be angry because I gave birth to a daughter . . . I had asked the doctor whether I had had a son or daughter. If a daughter, how would I return home? When I asked that, [my husband] scolded me."

Durga's husband and parents-in-law said nothing to her about giving birth to a second daughter. By her own admission, no one in her husband's family (*ghar*) had expressed disappointment that she had not yet produced a son, but she felt disappointed nonetheless. She had internalized the necessity for sons. When I asked Durga if she felt she needed a son, at first she said no. Later she admitted, "No, it would have been better if she (the second daughter) had been a son. Thinking that I would get a son, I gave birth [the second time]. I didn't get a son, and what can be done?" She made the point that she could not control the sex of her children, but nevertheless felt the disappointment of not producing a son. In the end, she concluded, "If I have [another child], then [it will be] much later, after they get bigger." Durga was twenty-seven at the time of that interview. Her daughters were aged seven and two. She felt that everyone was implicitly expecting her to have another child, yet she was reluctant to do so.

Sita (#135 wife of middle son) also expressed the necessity for having sons primarily in terms of her own internalization of that expectation. She had two daughters, at that time aged four and seven, and when asked whether she needed to have a son, she said, "I don't need one, but others disagree." Others, she said, meant her parents-in-law. "They say they need at least one." When asked about her husband's preferences, she replied:

> He doesn't need one. Now he says not to give birth. My husband says, "Why have many births? It will be alright if we don't have another birth." We are only two; because of others we are not able to [avoid giving birth again]. I practiced temporary family planning. I haven't adopted a permanent method. I feel that I don't know what to do. It is uncomfortable. It would have been so nice if the youngest daughter had been a son. It would have been carefree (*aananda*). No one would have been able to say anything. In our society, it is said that a son is needed; that isn't good. And also *Deuraani* (her husband's younger brother's wife) had a son; I had two daughters. When sisters and aunties came, they told me that they wanted to see one from me. Everyone that came [said that]! I couldn't do anything. What to do?

When asked what her husband thought after the birth of the second daughter, she assured me, "He didn't behave badly; he didn't. But I felt bad myself when I gave birth to a daughter in the hospital that time." Contradicting her earlier general comment that her parents-in-law needed a son, Sita said that her parents-in-law were supportive after the birth of her second daughter. Her parents-in-law told her that a daughter is just like a son and not to feel disappointment (*dukha*). But this statement was a consolation, not a negation of the need for a son. Even though no one in her family said anything negative to her about giving birth to a second daughter, she had internalized the expectation of a son. "I thought, 'What will others say because [I had] another daughter?' So I felt bad. But no one said anything. I felt bad myself." Although no one said anything, Sita felt unsatisfied. As with many expectations within Nepali families, there was no need to express aloud that which was already understood.

Toward the end of the interview, about an hour into my fourth discussion with Sita over a period of seven months, she contradicted her earlier statement that she did not feel the need to have a son: "I will see once. I will give birth once more. And if it isn't [a son], what to do, no? They told me to give birth. No one listens to me. What to do? I will try one more time. If again it is a daughter, then I will go to my *maaita*, have [the sterilization] operation there, and return. [I will do that] whether or not it causes my husband to marry another. It doesn't matter to me. I am thinking that now." This couple may have agreed on a philosophical level that they do not need a son, but on a more realistic level they felt the need for one. At that time, in 2004, Sita had said she would likely try for a son one more time despite having used Norplant® to avoid becoming pregnant for the past five years. She seemed to be testing the limits to the rules about producing a son, waiting to see what would happen and how bad the situation would get before she allowed the possibility of becoming pregnant again.

When I spoke with Sita again in 2009, she said that in fact the situation was similar. She and her husband did not mind that they did not have a son, but that her parents-in-law and even her own parents were dissatisfied with the situation. During our conversation that summer, which took place seated comfortably in upholstered chairs in her living room with some of her cousins, she reiterated that one of the main reasons why she should not give birth was because she thought her body was too weak. She had an ongoing problem of no appetite, but after not eating anything she feels weak and vomits. And indeed, Sita had been notably thin ever since I had known her. Upon hearing this, her elder cousin commented that before, in her time, such a weak wife would have been sent back to her *maaita* and the husband would have taken another wife. "But times have changed," the cousin said. It was left ambiguous whether her statement was one of support for Sita or a critique of her weakness.

Sita then brought up another point in support of her behavior, that there would be no "guarantee," using the English word, that the next child would be a son. Her elder cousin responded again, saying that these days people check the sex of the baby by doing an ultrasound, then abort it when they find out that it is a girl. Both the women quickly stated that they thought that practice is not good, that it is sinful. Sita said she refused to do such a thing, and therefore there is no "guarantee" of having a son. If she could be certain that she would get a son, she said, then she would give birth again. But since it was not possible, she would not. Later in our conversation, the elder cousin proclaimed that nowadays girls are just like boys. She said that they can become doctors, pilots, anything. Girls are just as good as boys. I agreed, but pointed out the one remaining difficulty described to me again and again over the years: girls move away when they get married and cannot care for their parents. The cousin politely agreed, the conversation awkwardly shifted to another topic, and I realized I had been a bit too brash in stating things so plainly.

Other women were more adamant about not giving birth again. They asserted that their daughters were just as good as sons. Radha, a twenty-four-year-old living with her husband and ten-year-old daughter (first introduced in Chapter one, HH #483), did not hesitate in responding to the question of whether she was interested in having another child:

> If [my husband] needs a son, then I will ask him to take another wife. After all, can we give birth to a son if we want one, or to a daughter if we want to have a daughter? If we have a daughter, [people's] behavior is so different; they insult. The very behavior of the family changes with the birth of either a son or daughter. So how can we have that? We are not machines. So what guarantee is there that my next child would be a son? Suppose I get only a series of daughters, then what? It will be very difficult to care for all the girls. We can't kill them, we have to look after them well, we have to earn a living. It is very difficult.

Radha summarized the observations of several young mothers living in nuclear families when she said, "Look at my own husband. He neither serves his parents in times of need nor cares for his wife. So I don't feel that a son is highly necessary. Instead, I feel that our daughter will give more love." Another woman living in a nuclear family remarked, "A son is no longer necessary. What have sons done in recent times? . . . If I can do well for my daughter, she too will take care of me. In the case of earning well, she too can do well." In response to her husband's opinion that girls are worth little and do not need to be educated, Radha conceded, "He is also correct in some ways, because a daughter is married off, whereas a son will be compelled to look after his aging parents."

Even the young women who were the boldest in their opinions could not dispute the fact that daughters leave their parents at the time of marriage. The patrilocal joint family system undermines the logic of women who said that having daughters is just as good as having sons. Women living in nuclear families hoped that their sons would stay with them and bring daughters-in-law into the household—recreating a joint family. Thus, although young women were dismissive of traditions related to their culture and religion, such as requiring a son to perform funeral rites, it seemed they could not escape their society's underlying assumptions about patterns of residence and marriage.

Conclusion

In Nepal, contemporary young mothers are positioned amid conflict-ing discourses of producing a son and the "small, happy family." While the women in this study claimed that religious explanations for needing to produce a son were fading, the multi-generational joint family ideal remained strong. Having (or expecting to have) a joint family household influenced women's desire for sons because they want to have a daughter-in-law to replace the daughters lost to other households through marriage. Despite resisting the necessity of sons and viewing daughters as capable and valuable, women were unable to escape the following: increases in the potential contributions of women to the household bene-fited them only through daughters-in-law, not through daughters. Young women's opposition to the high value placed on sons in their society ulti-mately did not overcome their desire for a daughter-in-law who would provide assistance and care. I have argued that the patrilocal extended family system thus continues to drive observed "son preference," despite the limitations of this term in capturing the characteristics of the situation (2010a).

The study of reproduction necessarily includes a consideration of the role of hegemony in reproductive lives (Greenhalgh 1995, 1990; Ginsburg and Rapp 1995) or the aspects of the body politic (Scheper-Hughes and Lock 1987) related to procreation, in this case ranging from the personal politics of women's relationships to the global politics of the messages and services of international population programs. Structural forces such as gender and reproductive norms are forces that may limit, but not dictate, the range of human behavior. Examining how people negotiate societal expectations through their relationships with others reveals how through the process of everyday dealings people manipulate, tear down, or rein-force norms and larger institutional frameworks (Bourdieu 1977; Ortner 1984). Young, married women's conflicted feelings about the necessity of producing a son are presented here within the context of fertility decline and the discourses surrounding it, sometimes with and sometimes against the older generation's explanations of the importance of having sons. Instead of the commonly repeated narrative of South Asian husbands and mothers-in-law pressuring young married women to produce a son, this research reveals a picture of women who, in this setting, have recognized the potential and limitations of daughters and the practical reasons behind the rhetoric of needing a son. Women acted pragmatically in matters of procreation within the sociohistorical circumstances, but all the while they proclaimed that they did not "need" a son.

The challenge in studying individuals and fertility behavior lies in "giving demographic actors agency without endowing them with a utility-maximizing rationality" (Greenhalgh 1995, 19). Reproductive decision-making, much like human agency, "is correctly understood not as a sequence of discrete acts of choice and planning, but rather as the reflexive monitoring and rationalization of a continuous flow of conduct" (Carter 1995, 61). Ultimately the "decision" to give birth in this research context is more a process than a moment, one that involves power dynamics between the sexes and among family members. Likewise, it is shaped by the structural constraints applicable to that context.

This research contributes an additional perspective on reproductive "decision-making": some women are using reproductive technology not to make a decision, but rather to stall. In a context in which they are facing conflicting discourses (one of which they seem to have embraced, while rejecting the other), son-less women are using contraceptives in an innovative fashion—to indefinitely delay giving birth again. The uncertainty of this "delay" could ultimately turn into the certainty of not ever having additional children. The success of this strategy—whether consciously employed or not—depends precisely upon the *lack* of a decisive move. Other scholars have concluded that *not* using contraceptives can be interpreted as a passive decision or a lack of decision that can lead to pregnancy. I argue that in a similar way, using contraceptives can accidentally lead to not having any more children. This type of stalling by son-less women is apt in a context such as this one: a patriarchal, patrilineal, and patrilocal society in which women who are in fairly comfortable living situations are wary of disrupting the family harmony.

Overall these are not stories of overt resistance against social expectations to produce a son. Social change is sometimes caused by such easily discernable actions, but more often it is a subtle, ongoing process. This account is an exploration of the latter. It is a mixture of both quiet and defiant voices. Some women voiced concern, ambivalence, and indecision, while others voiced clear frustration with the cultural and familial expectations placed upon them as women. These glimpses into the minutiae of women's reproductive lives and decision-making provide insight into social change of the more everyday variety, and captures—for a moment— the dynamic flow of the dialectic of culture and the individual. The reproductive bodies, beliefs, and behaviors of Nepali Hindu-caste women thus illuminate the gradual acceptance or rejection of new ideals and illustrate creative employment of new medical technologies.

In a scenario in which women are caught between contradictory discourses of smaller families and the importance of producing a son, reproductive behavior can be a process of trying things out—or even stalling—in order to test limits and options. Despite many verbal statements to the contrary, ultimately young, son-less women were unable to escape the need for a son and the ideal of the multi-generational joint family. Observing their teenage sons' behavior, however, a few women wondered aloud whether sons these days would actually be of any real value.

4

Son Preference and the Preferences of Sons

On a warm evening in July of 2009, I was zigzagging through the crowded, narrow backstreets of Kathmandu in a typical Maruti Suzuki 800 taxi with an overly energetic driver. I had returned to follow up with the teenage sons of the women I interviewed in Vishnupura in 2003–2005. The stereo of the diminutive car was blaring a song on repeat with the refrain, "I gotta feeling, that tonight's gonna be a good night." I did not recognize the song at the time, but the lyrics were indelibly entered into memory after the third time it was played at high volume. Only several months later did I hear the song back in the United States and search for its story.

"I Gotta Feeling" was the hit single from The Black Eyed Peas' album, *The E.N.D.*, released on May 21, 2009, and debuted on the Billboard Hot 100 the week of June 27, 2009. The song later reached number one on the U.S. charts and was nominated as Song of the Year at the 2009 World Music Awards. Worldwide, it became one of the most successful songs in the history of popular music. The Black Eyed Peas are an American hip-hop band, and it is notable that their song became a hit on a global scale so quickly that a taxi driver in Nepal was playing it only a few weeks after it climbed the charts. Globalization is not new and has been around for decades if not centuries. Moreover, Kathmandu has a distinct history as a gathering place for world travelers of a certain type: Europeans and Americans engaged in mountaineering and/or counterculture. The stream of hippie tourists of the 1960s and 1970s spurred the formation of entire neighborhoods in Kathmandu that cater to tourists, first Freak Street and more recently Thamel. However, such a *high speed* of global sharing that led to my embodied experience of globalization—being subjected to the thumping bass of "I Gotta Feeling"—appeared qualitatively different from that which I had observed in the Kathmandu Valley even within the previous decade. My interviews with young men in 2009 and 2010 bolstered this impression as we discussed their mobile phone models, favorite music, and clothing styles.

Young men and globality may, at first glance, seem like a surprising turn in a narrative of women and reproduction. However, following up with the sons of the women who I had originally interviewed in 2003–2004 was the next logical step after women explained to me how the need for a son was still a prominent feature of their family life and reproductive projects due to the patrilocal marriage system. If it turned out that sons were not going to fulfill their duties to their mothers and fathers, then the cycle of needing a son in order to gain a daughter-in-law in order to look after the family and its future interests would be interrupted.

During our conversations about the roles of daughters and sons in 2003–2005, several women turned their attention toward their own sons and laughed or despaired. They commented on how their sons were disrespectful, did not obey their parents, were absent for long periods with no explanation, and skipped classes at school or neglected their studies. A few used drugs or alcohol, dyed their hair blue, or wasted too much money on jeans (according to mothers). Observing their teenage sons' behavior, a few women wondered aloud whether sons these days would be worth the investment.

Five to six years after this initial research period during which women expressed these concerns, several sons of these women (and others like them in the community) were poised for major demographic and cultural events such as marriage. These young men and their peers grew up during the Maoist insurgency and came of age in a time of instability and dramatic social change. In 2009 and 2010 I conducted a follow-up study of their perspectives on post-monarchy "New Nepal," new technologies for building social and romantic relationships, and their attitudes toward marriage and caring for aging parents. The fundamental question motivating the research was, are these sons going to fulfill their duties to their mothers in the way that their mothers had imagined? Will the promises of a son—bringing a daughter-in-law into the household, providing care as the parents age—actually be fulfilled by the new generation of young men?

The final chapter of this research project asks if these young men's aspirations for their own union and procreation reflected a sense of individualized agency or a continued commitment to the joint family. Did they envision living in their fathers' households and perpetuating the joint family system? To whom or to what ideologies did they feel a sense of duty; or had the trope of duty been replaced by locating oneself within social relations in some other meaningful way? The significance of how these young men navigate the incursion of historic political and social changes as well as global trends reaches far beyond their own futures and those of their aging parents. Their decisions impact the continuation of the joint family system and son preference.

Coming of Age in a Historic Time

The cohort of young men in Vishnupura who in 2010 were poised for marriage had come of age during a tumultuous and eventful time in Nepal's history. When they were young children in the 1990s, Nepalis had agitated for an end to the king's absolute power in favor of a constitutional monarchy and a popularly elected, multiparty parliament. In 1990 the Nepali "people's movement" (*jana aandolan*) had ushered in a period of popular political participation previously unmatched in Nepal's history of Rana kings. The optimism for progress and freedom soon faltered, however, as successive elected governments proved to be ineffectual and corrupt (Liechty 2003). Though as children they were likely oblivious to these events, the cohort witnessed a somewhat similar set of events as teenagers and young adults: the overthrow of the constitutional monarchy due to the combined pressure of public protests by the political parties and their student counterparts and a communist insurgency by a group that labeled themselves the People's Liberation Army. This group is often simply referred to as *Maaowaadi* by the public, but technically is just one part of the Communist Party of Nepal (Maoist).

The beginnings of the Maoist People's War in Nepal can be traced to 1995, with the violence intensifying in 2001 in coordinated attacks on army and police posts in the western regions. After over 12,000 deaths and multiple false starts at a peace agreement, the government and Maoists signed a peace accord in 2006, declaring a formal end to the decade-long civil war. Maoist leaders joined the political mainstream, and Parliament approved the abolition of the monarchy in 2007. Nepal officially became a republic later in 2008.

The abolition of the monarchy was one of the major goals of the People's Liberation Army (PLA), but ostensibly so was a more just social system that would unseat high-caste Hindus and Newars from their dominant political, economic, and social positions in the country. The PLA also advocated for gender equity, incorporating women into their ranks as soldiers and support, but the extent to which gender equity truly was achieved is dubious (Brunson and Boeger n.d.). "*Nayaa* Nepal," or New Nepal, became the catchphrase for the state of the country in the wake of the ceasefire and formation of a new republic, and indeed initially many people were optimistic about the future of their country as a constituent assembly formed to draft a new constitution. But a series of clashes among politicians and subsequent resignations, one of the biggest in 2009 between Prime Minister Prachanda (the former leader of the People's War) and President Yadav over the integration of former Maoist rebels into the national army, combined with multiple missed deadlines for drafting the new constitution, dampened public spirits and hopes for a "new" Nepal.

The local community had undergone significant changes, as well, during the young men's coming of age. Land prices in Vishnupura skyrocketed, creating windfalls of cash for small-scale agriculturalists who sold their land. Local real estate brokers profited as well. The pace of development was palpable, with new houses popping up on the landscape at a steady rate and dirt roads being paved and new ones plotted. Entire neighborhoods sprung up as developers accumulated agricultural land, and as of 2012 even a trendy local organic farming cooperative had opened in one of the new neighborhoods. And, though at least since the 1980s Vishnupura has been a desirable place of residence for wealthy Kathmanduites and home to several imposing estates that stand out dramatically among more meager residences, it was increasingly becoming less an independent village and more a suburb of Kathmandu.

Besides all the new homes in Vishnupura, the other most notable change was the way people spoke about a loss of optimism about their country and their society. The daily newspapers contained headlines that announced the breakdown of the state and the greed of individuals both in government and civil society. Friends and shopkeepers chatting on the streets echoed these themes in their casual conversations. I overheard many versions of offhand comments about the uselessness of the government, and that "New Nepal" was merely an empty phrase. Several high-profile kidnappings had occurred recently, and they had captured the popular imagination and were inciting much discussion. People joked sarcastically about all the different groups calling strikes during those days; they could not keep up with what strike was when and who had called it. Friends warned me to be careful; hit and run accidents were common, and no one wore gold jewelry anymore for fear of someone driving by on a motorbike and yanking it off. The extent to which these concerns were "real" is beside the point; the fact that a pervading sense of lawlessness was expressed repeatedly by acquaintances and strangers alike, as well as in formal interviews, stood out from my past stays in Vishnupura and Kathmandu.

The coincidence of a thief coming to my Nepali family's house one night while I was there made these public discourses seem real enough. Everyone but my *bahini* (younger sister), who often stayed awake later than the rest of us, was sleeping, and she spotted a man climbing between the balconies of the close houses. The year prior, my adopted mother saw someone trying to access a neighbor's house with a ladder, and she threw a rock at him and scared him away. Apparently another neighbor had been robbed recently because both husband and wife worked during the day and the daughter went to school, leaving the house empty. A group broke into the house during the day as a result. This sparked a discussion of how at that time young men of low economic status had started receiving an education and therefore were embarrassed to do physical labor or menial jobs; consequently some resorted to stealing. Someone speculated that young former Maoists were also struggling and could not find jobs, so sometimes they resorted to stealing as well. These stereotypes are not repeated here as sociological truth or to endorse such views, but rather as a window onto people's assumptions at a time when society as a whole was anxious about such lawlessness.

I interviewed thirty-three young men living in Vishnupura, in small groups consisting of friends (after pretesting revealed that the young men talked substantially more when with a companion). Six of the young men were sons of the women I first interviewed in 2003, and the remaining participants were friends of theirs or young men of similar age from the community selected in an attempt to round out characteristics of the small sample such as education or socioeconomic status. I excluded individuals from the two extremes of the socioeconomic scale, the very wealthy and the destitute. It would be inaccurate to lump the participants together as "middle class," however, since some of the young men came from the upper range of middle-class families and attended private colleges, while others had dropped out of school at an early age in order to begin working. In this section of the book, I spend less time describing the participants in detail because several of the young men have characteristics that make them easily identifiable. Socioeconomic status and caste or ethnic identity were two aspects of identity that are indispensible in situating their comments, however, so I include those at the very least.[1] Unlike my interviews with women in their homes, these interviews took place in unoccupied corners or patios of modest local coffee shops, outdoors sitting on the ground in an expanse of forest popular with local young people, or in the common room of my Nepali family.

Overall, despite their youth, the men were quite articulate about all the changes happening around them. They discussed how the model of one's

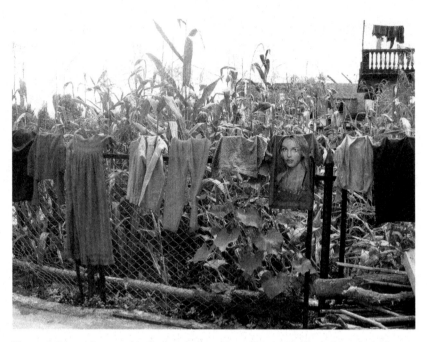

Fig. 10. A Britney Spears t-shirt hangs among more traditional Nepali clothing items, drying in the sun.

mobile phone had become an indicator of social status, how their favorite music and television shows had become a mixture of Nepali, Hindi, and English media, and they wore not just the mass-produced Britney Spears t-shirts that were available at bottom discount prices from roadside vendors (most likely shipped over land from bordering China, like many of the cheap manufactured goods available on the streets in Kathmandu), but also a Beatles shirt or stylish jeans that must have taken effort, intention, and sufficient cash to purchase. Despite the extended discussion of all that was changing, on one topic the young men's ideas did not sound different from their mothers': sons taking care of their parents.

Change and Similitude: Not-so-*Nayaa* Nepal, Gender Roles, and Patrilocality

Dev was seated on the forest floor in the shade of tall pines. We had gathered in this popular outdoor destination for young people (see Brunson 2014) with three of his friends, all of different castes or ethnic groups. Several of the young men had shoulder-length hair, but Dev kept his particularly neat, his waves framing his face. He was short by Nepali standards, but he had a noticeably muscular build, clearly the result of lifting weights. He wore a fashionable black t-shirt with a deliberately frayed applique and jeans. He spoke with a slight stutter.[2]

DEV (#2): So, you are a researcher and will write a book. What did you expect from us? Did we say what you expected?

JAN: There are so many changes for your generation, no? But one thing is the same. You all said that you will take care of your parents well in the future. I have noticed others saying the same thing.

DEV: This thing won't change. When we have children, they will also say the same thing.

Dev came to this conclusion after an hour-long discussion. At only nineteen years old, he summarized several aspects of social life in Nepal with the acumen of a social scientist, avoiding generalizations and pointing out the differences between the educated and uneducated, rural and urban populations, as well as how economic pressures drive certain behaviors. Dev's assertion that "this thing won't change," by which he means sons taking care of their parents, sums up what all of the young men reported to me about the persistence of the joint family ideal and the underlying assumption of patrilocality. So many things had dramatically changed in these young men's lifetimes, and yet so much had stayed the same. In this section I attempt to capture some of the subtleties and contradictions of several significant changes: not-so-new "*Nayaa* Nepal," radically different yet oh-so-familiar gender roles, and the persistence of patrilocality at the same time everyone was trying to go abroad.

Nayaa Nepal refers to the advent of a new phase in Nepal's history marked by the end of the constitutional monarchy and Nepal's royal family, and the beginning of a new republic and a new constitution. It also implies the replacement of the dominant status and practices of the Hindu high-castes with, at least hypothetically, a new set of social rules that value ethnic diversity. Nirmal and Abhi (Thakuri and Newar, respectively), two of Dev's friends, summed up the situation in this way:

NIRMAL (#2): Before, when there was a king, he was the "head." There was a compulsion to follow him, so everybody obeyed him. But now, there are Maoists; there are Limbuwaan (Limbu), Khambuwaan (Rai), Tarai Jana Mukti Morcha (refers to Tarai People's Liberation Front), Himaali (people of the Himalayas), PahaaDi (people of the hills). Everywhere, there is "competition." That's why there is no peace in Nepal. When there was king, it was not like this. Everybody had to follow him.

ABHI: (*overlaps*) Now there is competition among one another. Everybody thinks himself equally important. Nobody thinks himself less.

Nirmal continued on, saying that even when one of the political parties tried to accomplish something good, the others would undermine their efforts. Such behavior led to the political quagmire and seemingly endless delays in drafting a new constitution. Also commenting a few days prior on this situation, Sushil, a high-caste Newar from a modest economic background who was highly dedicated to his studies, explained:

> SUSHIL (#1): In 2006 there was one "movement," *aandolaan*, at that time there were politicians to teach [the people involved in the movement]. They, the politicians, taught us, "We have to make Nayaa Nepal," "We have to make Nepal a republic," "We have to remove the monarchy," no? Having elected them, we Nepalis sent them to the constitutional assembly, and now they have forgotten what they told the people. All are building their own houses, they are fighting for posts; they said Nayaa Nepal, but there was no politician who was for the people. Politicians/leaders were produced, and they went to fight for posts, and before even one year passes the government changes. Now again they have made a new government. In the newspaper it will say this government is a fabrication, it is fake government, it won't last more than two or three months. Those kinds of things come out. Only the name has changed.

For the majority of the young men I interviewed, the catchphrase "New Nepal," rather than signifying a new and promising time of democracy, in reality meant a continuation of "old" Nepal, with an added measure of lawlessness and economic inflation. BK, the son of Maya (whose story is told at length in Chapter two, HH #140), summarized it this way:

> BK (#5): During the time of the King, people did not violate the rules, so there was "freedom." Nowadays there are many crimes happening in the country like killing, fighting . . .

Later he added:

> BK: In the beginning, when "Nayaa Nepal" arrived, we used to be curious. At that time we discussed it a lot. But now, what is there to say—"Nayaa Nepal" and "Old Nepal" are the same! What is there to say?
>
> (*LAUGHTER*)
>
> BK: No change, so how can one call it "new"?

The phrase "Nayaa Nepal" had become a source of jokes and wordplay, as well as bitterness. Suresh, a twenty-year-old Tamang student, in response to the question, "What does Nayaa Nepal mean?" joked,

SURESH (#13): In front the word nayaa is added, otherwise nothing new.
    (LAUGHTER)
SURESH: There is a saying 'jun jogi aayepani kaanai chireko' (a well-known Nepali proverb meaning whoever comes is the same).[3]
Whichever political party comes, it is the same.

Another common joke was that Nayaa Nepal meant *aandolan*, which refers to a movement or protest, sometimes characterized by a general strike or closure (*bandha*) in which no traffic is allowed on the roads and shops remain closed. Prior to Nayaa Nepal the Maoists were responsible for calling most of the day-long or even multiple-day closures, but the young men claimed that in Nayaa Nepal almost any group would call for a strike. Several young men described how these closures had interrupted their submission of applications to study abroad, taking school exams, and even taking national level exams, for basically one cannot travel anywhere except places within walking distance for fear of violent retribution. For those depending on daily wages, such strikes could mean missing a meal.

Two economically disadvantaged young men, Gopal and Rajesh, both working as assistants to truck and bus drivers, conveyed the harsh reality of Nayaa Nepal for the laboring classes. At first there were four young men seated for this interview, but two quickly ran off after their boss called their cell phones to say they were needed to work.

GOPAL (#3): (*in a loud voice*) People say Nayaa Nepal, but thus far I have not seen anything new. Prices for everything are becoming high . . . This is Nayaa Nepal.
RAJESH: Unemployed people are still unemployed, and employed are working. Everything is the same. This is Nayaa Nepal. Vegetable prices are so high. Those who work, they get to eat; and those who don't work, don't get to eat.
GOPAL: These politics have increased the price of everything. It's becoming very hard to have even *daal bhaat* (the staple Nepali meal of rice, lentil soup, and curries).

Their frustration reveals the experience of the poor in a time of rising prices and few job opportunities. They indicated it was challenging to find a job, even for individuals willing to do less prestigious work like being a "conductor" (the assistant or fare collector, not the driver) on vehicles.

I will return to the situation of the laboring classes later in this chapter. Moreover, I will address the connections between political and economic insecurity and the preference for a joint family, and why all of these factors are intimately linked to women's projects of reproduction.

In addition to political change and lack thereof, young men discussed their thoughts on recent developments in gender roles and duties. There were similar themes of change and similitude, of novel and familiar gendered social proscriptions. The most significant aspect of young men's discussion of gender roles for my research was the fact that several young men brought up the topic of patrilocality long before I asked any questions about it in the interview. Prior to asking about gender roles, we had discussed music, mobile phones, social media, and politics—nothing that would prompt them to answer my broad question, "What are the differences in the roles and duties of girls and boys?" with responses about patrilocality. I argue, therefore, that the fact that they responded in this way highlights the social centrality that it occupies in people's reckonings of gender, as well as their assumptions about their futures.

Nirmal and Abhi, Dev's friends introduced above, described the differences in the roles and duties of girls and boys in this way while we sat together in the forest:

ABHI (#2): In urban areas, it (equality) is increasing. Although daughters are not equal to sons, it is improving. But, if we go beyond town areas, the girls are still carrying a *Doko*. The families think they will educate sons and will consider them as the family head. But they think they will send their daughters after marriage to another's house. In town areas, the daughters are to some extent equal. Maybe 25 percent of girls have equality in towns. But in villages, they are still dominated.

NIRMAL: The teenager son, who has not entered into the "practical life," thinks just of studying and having fun. But the girls think that they are grown up and they are of marriageable age. So, thinking that they cannot do anything (support) for family later (after marriage), they support the household work. They care for the family. But the boys eat, wander around, and have fun. They do not care very much about their family. That's the way it is.

ABHI: Obviously, there is a difference. Sons are considered the head of the family. In foreign countries, that does not exist. In the Nepalese context, the sons are still considered the heads of the family . . . and only they can do . . . Of course, after marriage, they have to manage the household activities. Daughters go (to other households) after marriage. They have two homes . . . but more responsibilities lie with the home she goes to after marriage because she has to spend her whole life there. Boys live in the same house after marriage. That's why they have to do for family. There is definitely a difference in responsibilities between boys and girls.

References to patrilocality permeated young men's discussions of gender and the differences between the duties of boys and girls. Several commented that these facts of life limit parents' willingness to educate girls. Their comments echoed similar thoughts expressed by women several years earlier regarding their daughters and the need for a son. Investing in a daughter's education was not a bad idea, according to mothers, but it would not benefit them; it would benefit the household into which the daughter marries. According to Shrimati's (HH #165) observations quoted in Chapter two, women also do not necessarily benefit from education or economic improvements if they are expected to do only household or agricultural work. Nonetheless, her family places great importance on education for their children, even consulting with me on one daughter's attempts to attend college in the United States. During my follow-up research with young men, Shrimati's son was away attending a residential medical college outside of the Kathmandu Valley. Manoj and I travelled to his college in order to interview him. He voiced similar misgivings about the impact of patrilocality on the chances of young women for education and careers:

> BIKKI (#9): In Nepali society, parents think that they want their sons to study well and take care of their parents during their old age. But for daughters, they want their daughter to be given to a good family and want her to fulfill her responsibility there in a proper way. I think they think that way. Parents want their son to do some good work in society. In Nepali society, the thing is, parents don't keep their daughter with them after they are 23 or 24, and I think that is the "big hindrance for development."

Rather than framing the issue in terms of gender equality, Maya's son, BK, points out that boys have greater roles *and* greater duties, possibly implying that with more power comes greater responsibility.

> BK (#5): Basically, boys have greater roles and duties than girls. You know, in our society, girls get married and are sent to boys' homes. For them (girls), their natal home becomes less "important." And furthermore, boys have to "handle" and take all the responsibilities of their family.

Typically sons are the ones sent out on errands for the family, whether to pay a bill or purchase a major item for the home, even if the task happens to be for his sister. Boys are trained to "handle" such family responsibilities prior to marriage. In sum, to quote Narayan (#13), "Boys have to take care of parents, but girls get married and go to their husband's house. So their duty and responsibility will be different."

Later in the interviews, when asked directly about whose responsibility it is to care for aging parents, young men responded with similar comments to those quoted above. The same explanation was told again and again, so to avoid redundancy I will use the succinct words of Niraj and Pradip. Both young men are Newar, but Niraj was slightly older at twenty-two years and was studying in college, while Pradip had attended school through grade nine.

> NIRAJ (#13): If a daughter cares for them, no problem; but in Nepal according to the culture, a son has to care for them rather than a daughter. Daughters are given to others. They think that way. Still, now, if a daughter is born they give priority to the son rather than the daughter.
>
> PRADIP: Parents will have expectations of their sons, and they try to give an education to the son rather than the daughter.
>
> NIRAJ: A son will care [for them], but a daughter is sent to husband's home. So.
>
> PRADIP: Daughters do not stay at their parents' [home]. They have to go to boys' homes and take care of boys' parents. That is all.

Only two young men mentioned that a nuclear family might also be good, as well, since that way there is no "tension" among family members. And a few young men qualified their intentions to live with their parents with statements that recognized there would be exceptions, such as if the family could not get along.

Thus while Nayaa Nepal initially promised a new beginning and fresh future for the nation, in fact the lived experience of it did not strike young men in Vishnupura as being that different. In fact, they noted several negative aspects of New Nepal, such as price increases and lawlessness. Likewise, while young men described the large difference in gender roles between women of their mothers' generation and their own female friends, they also emphasized how families continued to invest differently in sons and daughters because of the knowledge that daughters would be given away to other households. Patrilocality occupied a central part in people's construction of gender.

Enduring Commitment to the Family

These expressions of enduring commitment by sons towards their parents were not unreflective statements of a social norm. As young men explained why they desired to live with their parents, several predominant themes emerged. A conversation among four friends during our interview captures several of the themes echoed across interviews.

These four friends were some of the most articulate and ambitious young men I came across among the thirty-three I interviewed. They came from varied family backgrounds. Bikas's family was Gurung and had only lived in Vishnupura for a few years, renting an apartment. He was studying for his medical school entrance exams, with the aim of becoming a doctor. Sushil's family was high-caste Newar, and they also had rented an apartment in Vishnupura for only about five years. He was an athlete on the national team, and he was studying for his bachelor's degree. Suman was born in Vishnupura, and his high-caste Newar family was well-established in the community. They owned their own home. Likewise, Laxman was also born locally and lived in a home his Brahmin family owned, and was studying for his bachelor's. His family, however, did not own common goods such as a television, computer, or a motorcycle. Although the young men came from different economic backgrounds, they were all seriously pursuing college and postgraduate degrees. These four young men were so thoughtful and expressive in response to the interview questions that their group interview took almost three hours and had to be divided up into two evening sessions. Suman's sense of humor and entertaining quips kept the mood lively during our discussions, but unfortunately none of his jokes are featured in the following quotes.

In response to the question, "What is your most important responsibility?" Suman leads off with the response of family:

SUMAN (#1): . . . for me, my family is supporting me. "What can I do for my family?" is my responsibility it seems.

LAXMAN: In my opinion… Usually from childhood, father, our own family, takes care of us. "Obviously," after we can understand things, after we become capable, "obviously" we have to do for our family. "Personally," for me, in my life my first "target" is to keep my family happy. I have to fulfill that target.

SUSHIL: When talking about responsibilities, there are two things. One has to think about family, that is one responsibility; one has to take responsibility. Actually, my dad has already passed away, and because I am the eldest son I have to think about the household.

I have to think about my younger brother, my elder sister, and my mother. And when considering things other than family, I also think about what to do or whether I can do something for society. And going beyond that, for my country . . . because my specialty is being an athlete, I have to do something for my country; I have to earn international medals, that's what I think. That is one thing, but the main thing is thinking about one's own family. One's main responsibility . . . is one's family, mother, brother, sister—those who are present now.

BIKAS: In my opinion, I am a student, I am studying for medical degree, my "aim" is to become a doctor, no? With that in mind, my first responsibility is my education, and from my education after I make a "stable foundation;" I will support my family. I will keep being important for my family. There must be active participation in all of the family's activities. Maintaining prestige is one responsibility. One has to make a stable foundation for one's career; such responsibility is ongoing. And last, after building a foundation, then family.

Some of the predominant themes touched upon here include the societal expectation that eldest son will care for the parents, indebtedness to parents, and a desire for a secure future through studying and building a career.

Young men acknowledged the societal expectation for sons, typically but not always the eldest, to live with and care for parents. For example, the four young men introduced above stated:

SUSHIL: My mom is alone. And Nepali culture is that parents live with elder son, so I don't think I will separate from my one brother and mom. I will live in joint family . . . I have no desire to live with my wife separately.

SUMAN: Parents take care of us from childhood, so after marriage I will not live with only my wife. I will stay with my parents . . . My parents did their responsibility and now it's my turn. That's how I feel. That's why I will live in a joint family.

LAXMAN: I am the only son. So I can't live separately, no?

BIKAS: Though I am the youngest son I desire to live with my parents in a joint family.

And, certainly, young men's feelings of indebtedness to one's parents involved a sense of responsibility or obligation. However, many also hinted at their recognition of a different aspect—of repaying the care and love that parents give to children. Young men expressed something emotionally more complex than simply doing something that was required of them. For example, when during one interview the word profit was accidentally introduced in an attempt to further explain what was meant by the advantages and disadvantages to living in a joint family, Narayan Thakuri, Jethi's (HH #77) son, corrected the mistake in the interview question by saying that profit was the wrong word. He continued, followed quickly by statements from his friends,

NARAYAN (#6): We live with family not because of profit.
SARAD: There will be people to guide us.
SANDIP: We'll get help.
SARAD: We'll receive love for a long time.

There was a significant affective element to young men's statements about their desire to remain living with their parents, so I highlight that here in the hope that it does not get overlooked among the more utilitarian benefits.

The other two main themes in sons' explanations of the advantages of joint families were the ability of elders to guide and instruct junior family members and the economic support and security offered by the joint family.

SUSHIL (#1): There are no disadvantages when we live with family because we will be living with our own family. But there will be advantages in the sense that our elders can guide and take care of our children more than we do. Elders are better people to teach rules and regulations and to make a "perfect human being." Our seniors will know more than us, so seniors can give more to juniors, more than we can.

BIKAS: . . . From the perspective of "security," it will be beneficial also. Thinking that my family (future wife and children) will be under the guidance of my brother and parents as well, I can feel at ease. And as he said, the older generation can teach more traditions than we can. [Without the joint family] we would be struggling to establish ourselves, and wife would be at home alone. It is better to have joint family and be secure.

Notions of security included economic ones, but extended beyond the economic as well. Sons believed their parents could help them raise their children to be good human beings and offer guidance and companionship to them and their wives.

Deconstructing Duty and the Family

As I listened to the young men talk, I was surprised by the loyalty and sense of duty that they expressed toward their parents. To an outsider, it seemed incongruous with some of their other expressions of individualism and efforts to distinguish themselves from the previous generation. Slowly I came to realize that I was pleased by their desire to care for their parents.

> MANOJ (#13): When parents get old and cannot work, who should take care of parents?
> SURESH: We should look after them.
> NIRAJ: That is a son's duty. That's why we are saying that we will stay together.
> SURESH: There is no sense of being a son if we cannot help them.

As an ethnographer who typically works with women, I want to raise the issue of how easily these young men's expressed devotion to family can be interpreted in an uncritical fashion. The young men's preferences follow a dominant cultural script about how, in order to be a "good son" one takes care of one's parents. It is all too easy in the analysis of their responses to slip into tacit agreement with this perspective. Whereas if I had been listening to young *women* speak on the same issues—duty to family, prioritizing the good of the family over one's own wishes—I automatically would have filtered their talk through a critical lens that took into account the structural reasons for why they valued and believed what they did.

In the following paragraphs, I briefly address three aspects of social structure that significantly impacted young men's agency and their relationship to the joint family. First, I describe how the ideal of the joint family faltered among young men from laboring classes. Second, I explain the challenges nuclear families faced due to being on their own. And last, I point out that due to constraints of Nepal's economy, sometimes parents are caring for sons more than sons are caring for parents. In many ways, the joint family is an *ideal*, and therefore falls short of reality.

A glaring contrast existed between the responses of young men from the laboring classes and those of young men living in more comfortable economic circumstances. Take as a starting point Nirmal and Abhi's description of what they perceived to be the differences between their fathers' generation and their own:

> NIRMAL (#2): It has been only ten–twelve years since this "town" has started to change. In the past, in this town too, people used to eat what they had (locally). But, now, there is a lot of showy behavior.

Just to show, people do more than their capacity. For example, if a neighbor buys a motorcycle, another person, due to jealousy, also buys a motorcycle without taking into account his financial capacity. He does not think about what will happen later or what could he do with that money. They do just to show others.

ABHI: Motorcycles are not bought for the parents, but because of children's demands. Everybody has a desire to have a motorcycle after seeing others. But, they (the children) do not think about how it affects their family even though they are of an understanding age. A child, at any cost, wants to fulfill his demand. Otherwise he will be down among his friends . . . The people from this area, before, used to go to the forest to collect firewood and sell it in Asan (one of the oldest and most important bazaars in Kathmandu), and, in return, buy flour and eat *DhiDo*. That's what I have heard. Isn't it the case, during our father's time? In our generation, it is not like this. We don't have to struggle. We roam around and eat without doing any work.

Nirmal and Abhi focus on generational differences here, but in the process they reveal their own comfortable situations and ability to roam around without doing any work. Several other young men indicated that they were able to relax and enjoy the companionship of their friends, often even searching for something to do out of boredom. A few spoke of being "busy" as a desirable quality, something to which they aspired. In an economy that does not offer a sufficient number of jobs, young men of a comfortable economic background found themselves with excess free time, looking for some activity to serve as what they called "timepass," a way to pass the time.[4]

In stark contrast, Dhan, a soft-spoken twenty-one-year-old who fidgeted anxiously, answered a question about how he spent his free time by saying he bathed, washed clothes, and cleaned. When followed by an inquiry of whether he sometimes met with friends, Dhan simply replied, "Usually there is work." Dhan's parents had died when he was young, therefore he had not had an opportunity to attend school except through the second grade. He worked in a small-scale furniture factory and lived with his two brothers in a single rented room, owned by the same family who owned the furniture factory. Though Dhan's situation was particularly dire due to the loss of his parents, I came across several such young men who left their parents and migrated at least temporarily to Vishnupura in search of agricultural or other such work. For some young men, their parents were not able to support them and they had to leave home searching for income. Thus in order for a joint family to function in a supportive role, even for young, unmarried sons, it had to have a certain level of economic capacity.

Nuclear family households comprise a sizable proportion of overall households in the joint-family system found among Hindus in Nepal and northern India. In a fertility regime in which producing multiple sons is the norm, at any given point one can find more nuclear families than joint families without negating the joint family as the overarching system and ideal. According to my survey of a representative sample of households in Vishnupura, married sons break off and form new households when the number of members in the stem family outgrows its ability to support them or the home runs out of space, there is discord between family members, there is a need to migrate to find work, to flee the violence caused by the Maoist insurgency, and to elope in an unsanctioned marriage.

Though lack of economic capacity may be a cause for children to leave their parents, tough economic times may also result from forming a nuclear family after marriage. In a joint-family system, young couples are absorbed into the larger economic unit of the multi-generational family and provided with a cushion that helps reduce the costs of housing, sustenance, and childrearing. In Vishnupura, living in a nuclear family was often characterized by economic hardship. Assuming that the split from the stem family was an amicable one, a son and his wife may claim some of his inheritance, but will be unable to depend upon the stem for additional major financial support. Moreover, most of the son's inheritance is typically tied up in land and therefore inaccessible. A common reason for an amicable split was to migrate to an urban area in search of a better income. If the separation results from a fight or disagreement, the resulting nuclear family undoubtedly will be in financial difficulty because a dependable cash income is difficult to come by. Therefore, rather than splitting from the stem family, sons often rely upon the wealth, the home, and agricultural output or income of their parents in an economy that cannot support enough wage-paying jobs. In my case studies of families, all the women living in nuclear households were engaged in income-generating activities: agricultural labor, sewing, cleaning, or working in a small shop.

Last, though the dominant discourse among these young men was that they would care for their parents, it should not be assumed that living at home in a joint family automatically means a son is a productive family member and is actually caring for his parents. A similar observation led Vera-Sanso to assert that sons live with aging parents; aging parents do not live with sons. It is incorrect to assume that young people are the ones doing the supporting in a joint family. Caring for aging parents is fraught with real-life complications, including the inability to care for them, as well as much less-common cases of neglect. Vera-Sanso also points out that a man's first obligation is down the filial line, to wife and children, rather than up it to parents. She concludes that a large number of aging parents in

India suffer from what she calls "intermittent childlessness," or the oscillation between periods of receiving some practical and/or financial help and periods of self-reliance (2004, 102).

Overall, young men in Vishnupura confirmed that being a good son was still defined as dutifully taking good care of one's parents. Despite their mothers' doubts about their dependability, young men professed intentions of returning the love and support that had been provided by their parents. These young men also demonstrate that duty is a two-sided coin. Their agentive commitment to "family" and their parents is, at the same time, at least a partial submission of their individual desires and opinions for what they perceive as the greater good. Their sacrifices for family result in benefits from the family.

Young men were limited by scarce economic opportunities in their nation, but they benefitted from the joint family system. In fact, their comments explicitly related the two. All of them reflected on the challenges for young men of standing on one's own feet; but their responses to this predicament varied. Young men from meager financial backgrounds in which their parents could not offer assistance were struggling in the best ways they knew how. Dhan was trying to work as many hours as he could in the furniture factory, and Laxman was working to better his position through education. Others from more financially comfortable households admitted that they were able to depend on their parents for their basic needs and were more concerned with "timepass" than anxieties about financial hardship. But even the latter group was responding to the frustration of insufficient job opportunities. Financial as well as affective reasons encouraged young men to remain in their comfortable joint families if at all possible.

Conclusion

In retrospect, I should not have been surprised to find these young men pronouncing the benefits of living with one's parents after marriage. Their most sought-after possessions—motorcycles, mobile phones, and other conspicuous symbols of class—were not obtainable from their own salaries, after all. Joint families offer an economic buffer for young couples who do not have reliable sources of income, and they can assist in shouldering the burdens of childcare and housework. Men maintain a privileged position in joint families in contrast to nuclear ones; in the latter they must take on many more responsibilities and yet share their authority more equally with wives. Furthermore, the young men expressed an awareness of the world moving around them—the fleeting trends of clothing and even politicians—and a desire to stay grounded through living with parents who can offer wise advice, teach traditions, and raise a new generation of "good human beings." Their experience of social vertigo inclined them to turn to their parents for much more than economic support.

The ideal of the joint family breaks down, however, under economic pressure when parents cannot adequately provide for their sons and their sons must migrate to search for work instead of completing their educations. And the extent to which sons really take care of their parents is also up for debate. But overall, if we return to the young men's mother's generation, and the rhetorical question that several of the women posed in the past, "Will these sons really care for us?" the answer, at least based on the young men's intentions, seemed to be yes. The remnants of what is labeled "son preference" in the social science literature—the desire to produce one or more sons to provide support as parents age—seemed to still be borne out in the preferences of sons.

5

Conclusion

Projects of Reproduction

The Hindu-caste women with whom I worked were not "planning" their families, for the concept of planning is tied too closely to the assumptions of Western notions of modernization and progress, assumptions they did not share. I suspect the application of the word planning to women's reproductive projects is inaccurate to varying degrees in many societies, in fact, for it implies too much control, predictability, and calculation. Sex, pregnancy, birth, and even marriages are notorious for not conforming to plans. Moreover, political economy influences the extent to which women have access to the logics and technologies of family planning (Maternowska 2006). And yet, Nila Chatterjee and Nancy Riley (2001, 815) describe how the modernist faith in humans as "rational, autonomous individuals who can control their environments and shape their own futures" is fundamental to the idea of family planning. Heather Paxson (2002) calls family planning advocates' attempts in Greece to promote a subjectivity of rational calculation and maximizing personal interests an attempt at "rationalizing sex." Furthermore, Lauren Fordyce (2012) demonstrates how quickly behaving "rationally" in one's reproductive life becomes moralized. Reproductive behavior deemed irrational, such as a so-called unplanned or unintended pregnancy, becomes labeled irresponsible or even immoral in a regime in which families ought to be planned. While governmental, international non-governmental, multilateral, bilateral organizations were all planning families in Nepal, Nepali women were engaged in something more subtle, complex, constrained, and dynamic than "planning."

In this book, I argue that reproduction is better understood and analyzed as a set of local and global "projects." Projects of reproduction imply actors who have desires, actions that have constraints, and an extended temporal aspect, for projects do not happen all at once. Projects are designed, abandoned, constructed, delayed, revised, interrupted, and remodeled over time. They are never truly finished or achieved, though eventually procreative capacities wane and death finds us all. A focus on projects risks an overemphasis of the power and intentionality of an individual over context and constraints (Ortner 2006), so I emphasize below how projects take place within structural limitations and in fact depend upon relations with others.

The term projects of reproduction also allows for the fact that they occur on different scales. A project of reproduction such as global fertility decline is launched on a global scale, though it surfaces in local languages and settings such as the posters described in the Introduction. Such global projects were born of the framework of progress that numerous scholars have critiqued (Tsing 2000), specifically in relation to fertility (Greenhalgh 1995; Chatterjee and Riley 2001), and more broadly in relation to development (Scott 1999; Ferguson 1997; Pigg 1992) and gender (Mahmood 2005). Large-scale projects such as population control are subject to historical events and milieus, and not unlike individual projects, they evolve over time. Rationales for projects shift as certain political positions come in and out of fashion, such as population control versus reproductive health (McNicoll 1995). They are altered to fit the latest buzzwords and ideals of the global development industry, such as reproductive rights or women's autonomy.

My articulation of projects of reproduction is based on what I observed unfolding over time on multiple scales, but it was inspired in part by Anna Tsing's discussion of how to study master narratives like modernization as social and historical artifacts (2000). Doing so is to "attend to the social practices, material infrastructure, cultural negotiations, institutions, and power relations through which modernization projects work—and are opposed, contested, and reformulated" (Tsing 2000, 329). Tsing was describing the ability of social scientists to study modernization as "a set of projects with cultural and institutional specificities and limitations" (2000, 328), in effect shedding modernization-think, and thus avoiding assuming the framework of progress that, in fact, generates the very concept of modernization. Rather than obliquely referring to some vague force such as modernization or globalization, relationships, pathways, and contexts need to be specified. I apply this approach to the way that discourses about planning families travel around the globe and mingle in local places and manifest in personal relationships. And I conclude by reflecting on how the notion of "progress" is not the only form of Western bias in discourses on health and development in the global South that deserves to be interrogated; freedom, often appearing in the guise of choice, does as well.

The Significance of Motion, or Merging the
Intersectional and the Dynamic

As stated in the Introduction, a motif of motion emerged from my interviews with women over time. Motion and a state of flux were also part of my analysis due to the longitudinal nature of this research. While intersectionality is critical for understanding women's diverse experiences, it does not adequately capture the flux of human intentions, actions, and meanings over time. Reducing women to a synchronic set of identity and demographic characteristics that correlate with their actions is insufficient (not to mention potentially dehumanizing or Orientalizing). Intersectionality is essential, yet not enough. It is essential in order to uncover the diverse experiences within a group falsely construed as similar, such as "Nepali women," but an intersectional analysis is unable to capture their creative negotiation of discourses on how they ought to act.

I devote an entire chapter to the significance of an intersectional approach in this research because an individual's position at the intersection of a variety of power axes is a vital consideration. Different facets of identity such as ethnicity, class, and gender can interact in surprising ways in different cultural contexts. Within a historically privileged group such as high-caste Parbatiya Hindus in Nepal, it is easy to overlook how class or other aspects of identity impact women's opportunities and constraints differentially. In this particular case the dominant social group also happens to have a reputation for the strictest gender rules regarding women's movement and behavior, due primarily to the perceived need to protect women's sexuality and prevent them from polluting others. High-caste women rank high on a social status hierarchy, but low on a hierarchy of gender power. Add a third power hierarchy, however, such as class, and assumptions about the status of such women start to fail.

In this book I have argued that ranking high in one prestige system and low in another prestige system can shape or challenge constructions of gender in interesting ways. For example, in this research, economic hardship acted as an equalizing mechanism for women of different castes, in some ways releasing women from the gender restrictions of their high caste, but at the expense of conditions that come with economic security such as a more comfortable life with fewer injuries and illnesses and less malnutrition. I illustrate the tradeoffs in different situations for women in which certain aspects of their well-being may be forfeited or suppressed while others are gained or improved. It is difficult to place a value on these different aspects, and therefore hard to compare them or come up with a net loss or gain. More specifically, I question the utility of measures of women's status such as autonomy because of their inability to capture these concomitant gains and losses in well-being. In order to capture these nuances and reach these conclusions, an intersectional approach was essential.

At the same time, an intersectional approach is insufficient for the following reasons. First, while it is absolutely critical to consider the structural limitations on women's behavior, it is insufficient to use structural explanations alone. This is hardly a novel statement in anthropology; since the so-called "postmodern turn" in anthropology in the 1970s, anthropologists have argued for the importance of studying agency, resistance, and social change, and rejecting overly deterministic portrayals of social structure. A balanced approach to studying social life does not overemphasize or romanticize women's agency, nor does it fail to recognize their potential for creative responses to structural constraints. And while intersectional analysis accounts for the complexity of identity roles in a woman's life, for many theorists it feels a bit too structure-heavy (Thompson 2007).

Second, women's projects develop over time. Goals may shift or diminish as contexts change or events unfold, and new significances may arise. In Ortner's words, "The intentionalities of actors evolve through praxis, and the meanings of the acts change, both for the actor and for the analyst" (1995, 175). In light of this quality of human behavior, an intersectional approach seems too static.

Demographic theories of fertility did no better at recognizing this quality of reproductive behavior. Susan Greenhalgh described how demographic theories of fertility tended to imagine that fertility decisions, or planning one's family, happen at one point in time, with perhaps a few minor adjustments after that (1995, 22). As a corrective, "anthropological students of family demography have reconstrued reproduction as an ongoing social and political construction that may begin long before and continue long after the biological fact of parturition" (Greenhalgh 1994, 5; compare with Jeffery and Jeffery 1997; Bledsoe 2002). Carter (1995) made significant strides in understanding reproductive decision-making, as demographers typically call it. Heralding his contributions, Greenhalgh writes that Carter "interprets human agency not as a sequence of discrete acts of choice and planning, the standard view, but as a reflexive monitoring and rationalization of a continuous flow of conduct, in which practice is constituted in dialectical relation between persons acting and the settings of their activities" (Greenhalgh 1995, 19).

Thus a preferable approach to understanding projects of reproduction would be one that could handle both the insights provided by intersectionality as well as by long-term, in-depth research. Life is always in motion. Synchronic snapshots can be useful, especially when comparing two or more of them, but I long for a methodology that can handle motion adequately. Perhaps the insights of Anne Marie Mol (2003) on the body multiple are useful in respect to reproduction. She conducts an ontological analysis of the different versions of reality and the work involved in making them cohere. Instead of multiple bodies, in my research there seemed to be multiple fertilities: fertility decline described by demographers, contraception acceptance rates displayed by Nepal's family planning offices, various iterations of the "small, happy family" message of the Family Planning Association of Nepal, and the complex combination of hopes for familial relationships, health, and security by married women engaged in reproduction. My observations resonate with the theory of another anthropologist, as well, who frames things quite differently but who also ruminates on the essentialness of motion in understanding social change in an age of globality. In *Friction*, Anna Tsing (2004) describes the process through which global and local groups talk about the environment yet speak of different things. Friction, she writes, is the result of these different groups engaging discursively, yet their words and ideas skid and deflect off one another as they pass/come into contact. And specifically in respect to reproduction, Charis Thompson (2007) attends to ontology, time, and shifting states. Addressing the high-tech side of reproduction, she calls the coordination of matters impending on what occurs in assisted reproductive technology clinics "ontological choreography." This type of coproduction of a "long-range self" (2007, 204), by reproductive technologies and doctors as well as the women in question, also has relevance for my story of low-tech reproduction and contraceptives. But while Thompson focuses on transformation that ARTs bring as a woman may become pregnant, I describe the details of maintenance of and by son-less women and their efforts to remain not-pregnant. These three ethnographies exemplify a turn towards motion as an underlying fundamental aspect of social theory and the promise of theoretical developments that can accommodate globality and flux.

Towards a Methodology of Projects

By paying attention to projects of reproduction as they unfold over time, novel and otherwise imperceptible strategies become discernable. Based on my ethnographic evidence, I have argued that stalling can be an effective strategy when women are faced with options they do not like, and I will expand upon the significance of this below. With the benefit of the hindsight that longitudinal research offers, I can also demonstrate how the strategy of biding one's time differs from stalling, and how the two reflect very different affective and economic contexts of marriage and childbearing.

As I describe in Chapter three, it was the women who did not have sons who offered the best insight into how women were negotiating social expectations and what the social repercussions might really be for women who refused to have additional children in order to try for a son. This was especially true for women with two daughters, for they had reached the "small, happy family" ideal of replacement fertility promoted by family planning organizations, but they had not fulfilled the social expectation of producing a son. They were caught between conflicting discourses simply due to the coincidence of giving birth to girls.

Sita's story, much of it summarized in Chapter three, is exemplary in its ability to advance a theoretical understanding of agency, resistance, and self-assertion. I define agency as the constrained capacity to act, following Sherry Ortner's (1984) and Laura Ahearn's (2001a, 2001b) interpretation of Bourdieu, and resistance as an explicit attempt to alter existing social relations or structures of power, following Michel-Rolph Trouillot (1995). One might use a term such as self-assertion to describe a milder version of resistance that is confined to maximizing one's position within a social system rather than changing it, or perhaps chipping away in barely perceptible increments at an existing institution, or even without intention causing small changes in larger power relations while focusing on one's own social relations and subjectivity. Sita never presented herself as resisting the social expectation to produce a son. Rather, she vacillated in her opinion on whether she should try again for a son, weighing the input of her husband, her in-laws, and members of her family's social circle in the community. In our conversations, her position on procreating a third time showed up as indecision. However, if one reads her actions rather than her words, by using Norplant, a contraceptive technology that only requires initial implantation in order to provide effective hormonal contraception for up to five years, she had taken a meaningful step towards not becoming pregnant. She was the only person in the case studies using Norplant, in fact the only case I had heard of among my general acquaintances. This is significant given that Norplant is the longest-acting temporary method of contraception available for women. Effectively what she was doing was stalling, or maintaining the status quo, and leaving her options open for the future.

The word stalling, though, has the potential to inaccurately imply inaction, so I must emphasize that Sita and others were actively seeking and using contraceptive technologies in order to delay becoming pregnant again. Most typically for women in this community, and in Nepal as a whole, such stalling would require a visit to a local clinic or sub-health post for a *dipo* shot (depo-medroxyprogesterone acetate, known in the United States by the brand name DepoProvera) every three months. Thus many women in Vishnupura were actively managing the prevention of pregnancy, taking their yellow cards and walking to the local health office every three months to receive the *dipo* injection. The one-room clinic was located upstairs from the local government office, and the line for *dipo* shots, available on designated days, extended out the door onto the veranda overlooking the small courtyard. Arriving and waiting at the clinic was hardly a private affair, as were the bright yellow shot records, as one woman who had attempted to hide her use of *dipo* from her husband informed me.

Stalling, or maintaining the status quo of not becoming pregnant, can eventually develop over time into a final outcome of having completed one's family size many years prior. If one stalls long enough, interested parties may abandon influencing one's procreation and pressures may decrease. And in Sita's case, as her daughters grew older, the idea of having a baby seemed increasingly peculiar to her and her family. The longer she stalled, the easier and more effective stalling became. In a reversal of the way that demographers discuss the failure to use contraception as becoming pregnant through inaction, I argue that stalling through using contraception can lead to completed fertility.

I first observed a similar strategy to "stalling," as I define it above, in women's explanations of why they were using temporary methods of contraception in a different time and setting in the Kathmandu Valley, in Kirtipur in 2000. Several married women who had two sons and were using temporary contraceptives explained to me that two sons were necessary, due to the possibility of one's young son becoming seriously ill, injured, or even dying. They used the saying, "One eye, what eye? One leg, what leg?" Meaning, what good is one eye, or one leg?[1] So after having two sons and completing their desired family size, they used temporary contraceptives rather than a permanent sterilization method in order to ensure their sons grew up healthy, capable, and productive. They were preserving their reproductive capacity just in case. I called this maintaining a holding pattern of fertility. While that was a very small convenient sample of women from clinics, my observations reflected national trends in fertility—historically in Nepal, initially temporary methods were not used for spacing, but rather after fertility was completed. Gradually this usage shifted towards more use of temporary methods for spacing between births as governmental programs began emphasizing birth spacing (Ministry of Health and Population et al. 2002).

Much had changed between then and five to ten years later, and women in Vishnupura claimed they only needed one son. And son-less women were in a more precarious position than the Kirtipur women with two sons back in 2000. However, there was some similarity in the use of general, somewhat passive, wait-and-see approaches, which I observed as a common strategy in non-fertility related matters as well. An acute and more extreme version of this is an action called *almal garnu*, when one causes confusion and/or delay in order to avoid doing or deciding something one would rather not do. For example, when it comes time to bid someone goodbye or to depart, a person may find excuses to delay the inevitable. What son-less women were doing was conceptually distinct from *almal garnu*, however, for their projects of reproduction extended over years in duration, and they were not attempting to generate confusion.

While perhaps a general tendency towards wait-and-see strategies can be observed in different facets of life, stalling as I define it above was employed in specific conditions. Stalling was a particular strategy employed in comfortable environments, economically and affectively. Other projects of reproduction were conducted in dire circumstances. The benefits of longitudinal research and hindsight allow me to assess Radha's case in retrospect and demonstrate how her strategy of waiting was distinct from Sita's. I realized from the outset of our conversations that Radha's case was sociologically dissimilar from Sita's: Radha was Dalit and had a meager education and income, she had married young after becoming pregnant, and she reported that her husband regularly partook of alcohol and other women. Radha was one of the most outspoken of the women in the case studies when it came to her refusal to produce another child despite having only one daughter, and it was clear that she was unhappy with her living situation. What I did not realize, however, until I discovered it in 2009, was that she would leave her husband. I tried to arrange a conversation with her husband or his relatives through a mutual acquaintance, but they refused to see me and would not provide any information on her where-abouts or how to reach her. Looking back, I realized that Radha was biding her time during the years that I knew her. Eventually she reached a point where she was either pushed past a threshold of violence that she deemed critical (Brunson 2011), or a particular opportunity to leave arose (for divorced women were highly stigmatized and had few options for living as a single woman or remarrying), or some combination of the two. Radha's case was also an example of how unpredictable reproduction can be. Her story involved an "unplanned" pregnancy in a rather extreme sense, since it occurred outside of a sanctioned marriage, and her project of reproduc-tion will continue to be shaped by these events as she moves forward.

Whereas Sita was stalling in her production of a son in a socioeconomic and familial context with which she was generally content and wished to maintain, Radha was biding her time to find out whether a way out of a marriage characterized by violence and infidelity would materialize. Son-less women were not willing to abandon or threaten a comfortable family situation, and women across all the case studies reported that the har-mony of family was the most significant determinant of their happiness. In this one exception, Radha's socioeconomic and family context became so untenable that she left. Projects of reproduction involve pragmatism, but that pragmatism looks different depending on the political economic and affective context of the woman.

Though these examples of son-less women make significant contributions towards a theoretical understanding of projects of reproduction, I now need to turn to the last piece of the overarching storyline of this book: why (and whether) sons matter. Even women who denied the necessity of sons ultimately concluded they were needed in order to bring a daughter-in-law into the family. And it was the sons who had the potential to break this family cycle if they decided to abandon the tradition of the joint family.

The Joint Family: Place of Refuge, System of Domination

Even the young women who were the boldest in their opinions about not needing a son could not overcome the social fact that daughters leave their parents at the time of marriage. The patrilocal, joint family model of living undermined the logic of women's statements that daughters were just as good as sons. In order to gain a daughter-in-law in the household in this family system, women had to produce a son. Women living in nuclear families hoped that their sons would stay with them and bring daughters-in-law into the home—transforming the household back into a joint family. So even though young women were dismissive of traditions related to their culture and religion such as needing a son for funeral rites, they couldn't escape social patterns of residence and marriage.

Women looked at their teenage sons, though, and wondered whether their unruly sons would in fact remain living with them, care for them as they aged, and bring a good daughter-in-law into the home. And as described in Chapter two, women did not necessarily think today's daughters-in-laws would make the mother-in-law stage of their lives much more comfortable than the previous stages. Today's daughters-in-law were too educated and worldly to shoulder the hard work of taking care of a home, garden, and perhaps a few animals, let alone agricultural work. These misgivings about upcoming generations had the potential to disrupt the joint family system.

Follow-up research with their sons and peers four–five years later (2009–2010) revealed conclusions that were surprising in light of women's fears, and not-so-surprising given the larger context of the benefits for young men of the joint family and patrilocal marriage system. Despite their attention to the endless parade of new fashion, music, and gadgets, the young men with whom I spoke in Vishnupura espoused views about family values that sounded remarkably similar to their mothers' generation.

In explaining why they intended to live with their parents after marriage, they referred to both the economic security and social or affective sanctuary that living in a joint family brings. They expressed a strong sense of deference towards their parents regarding family values and knowledge of what is morally right and of value in life. Among them, however, the most destitute young men were too focused on their current employment and daily living to reflect on such lofty concerns. Additionally, some of them had migrated to Vishnupura from surrounding rural areas looking for work, and they did not intend to return to their villages because of the lack of jobs in those locations. Therefore the idea of returning to live with their parents seemed unlikely.

The explanation of the persistence of son preference (and the joint family and patrilocal marriage systems) is not only a story of mothers and the sex of their babies, male or female; it is also a story of what sons want. Without sons advocating for staying with their parents, other effects of modern life could easily sway patrilocal practices. And in the case of the most destitute, perhaps it always has—whether sons from remote areas migrate to Vishnupura to find work, or from Vishnupura to Qatar or Saudi Arabia. But middle-class sons think they need the support of their parents, financially and affectively, in order to secure a comfortable life. The refuge of the joint family helps mitigate a meager economy, political instability, and anxious futures. Sons expressed this to me, but I also observed it first-hand in the differences between the joint family and nuclear family households and their histories in my case studies. The desire to remain in a joint family effectively perpetuates limits on women's choice to have only daughters and the ability of daughters to be sufficient to take care of their parents.

Pathologizing Patrilocality, the Undesirability of Freedom, and the Fallacy of Choice

In sum, the logic of my argument is as follows. Despite notable increases in women's education and perceived capacity to contribute to society through professional means, women in Vishnupura still felt they needed to produce a son to help secure their own future well-being through the presence of a daughter-in-law, due to the persistence of the joint family and patrilocal marriage, which is perpetuated by sons' desires to remain in joint families. In this logic, patrilocal marriage becomes the obstacle in the way of progress towards gender equity. In effect, patrilocality is pathologized as something that is bad for women's well-being. In closing, I would like to unsettle the last step in this logic: that patrilocal marriage is constraining women's reproductive projects, and more broadly, their overall well-being. This statement is both true and untrue.

In some ways it is true. If one analyzes societies around the world in a comparative fashion, the ones with patrilineal kinship and patrilocal marriage practices are also more restrictive of women's behaviors (Das Gupta 1995). And in societies that practice patrilocal marriage, women who marry farther away from their natal families are at greater risk for mistreatment than women who marry nearby or in their own villages (Dyson and Moore 1983; Niraula and Morgan 1996; Tan and Short 2004; Bossen 2007; Brunson 2011). Thus I feel justified in concluding that the patrilocal marriage system limits or constrains women's reproductive projects, and even more so because women directly stated this to me. I cannot claim credit for making that conclusion on my own.

But the above statement is also untrue, or at least flawed. Taking a social practice such as where one lives after marriage and assigning it a negative status because of its correlation with a trait deemed undesirable (in this case son preference, or constraints on the reproductive projects of women) relies on an underlying narrative of progress. The unspoken assumption in such logic is that women's equality with men is a valued, shared, and perhaps even a universal goal, and that evidences of gender inequities such as son preference are social problems that need to be fixed. I have reflected critically on such narratives of progress throughout this book, citing a list of scholars who have challenged modernization theory and even progressive notions of gender equality (Mahmood 2005). As Stacy Pigg and Vincanne Adams observed, "Questions of human rights, social justice, and survival, even when articulated in a self-consciously anticolonial manner, are usually tethered to the visions of progress inherent in secular liberalism, capitalism, and science" (Pigg and Adams 2005, 13).

Ultimately I am sympathetic to both sides of this argument, for both make good points. Nevertheless, here is one solid contribution I can make to this complex issue: improvements to women's well-being should not be grounded in their "freedom" or their ability to "choose." This ethnography, in which women's and sons' life projects are inextricably part of their relationships with family members, is a keen example of why that particular narrative of gender progress is illogical. Regarding freedom, in Chapter four I discuss how familial relationships are a two-way street. Family members benefit from those relationships as well as defer to and prioritize others' needs to meet the concomitant obligations that go hand-in-hand with the benefits. Why should women's freedom be a primary goal, when freedom would signify an absence of social relationships necessary for their well-being as social beings? Being socially untethered is akin to being outcast. As social beings, we are dependent upon those ties. Family relationships bind and chafe, but they also have the potential to soothe, protect, and cushion. And when they become too abusive, such as in Radha's case, it is imperative that one is able to attempt to find new "family," whatever unconventional form it may take, such as group homes for women (a strategy that many local NGOs have instituted). Or as in Maya's case, when her mother-in-law's restrictions became unbearable, the nuclear family breaks from the joint family, even though it causes serious financial insecurity. In this way, relations that are mutually supportive are the end goal, not freedom.

The notion of "choice" has equally troubling flaws. Arguments that focus on increasing women's choices as a means to improve their well-being fail to recognize that unmitigated freedom for women does not exist. Women may make choices, but those so-called choices are constrained by the conditions of inequity in which they live. Unequal power relations—whether related to gender, or compounded by another aspect of identity such as ethnicity or caste—are a precondition to any choice a woman makes. Pamela Stone (2008) demonstrates this perfectly in her rebuttal of the common narrative that women in the United States choose to leave their jobs to stay home and raise their children. She argues that such a claim completely overlooks the structural inequities that led women to make that choice: insufficient state support for paid parental leave and childcare, among others. Stone concludes that these women did not opt out of their careers; they were pushed out. This is the fallacy of choice.

With these points in mind, I offer a word of caution about the recent trend in celebrating women's reproductive "choices." As the dominant global narratives moved from constructing "Third World" women as fertile objects that had to be targeted in order to avoid global overpopulation, to constructing women as neoliberal, agentive individuals responsible for choosing small, happy families, are women any less subject to hegemonic discourses? On the surface, moving from a position of fertility control tinged with eugenic motivations, to one of reproductive health and human rights that espouses women's equality and empowerment, would seemingly be a positive (or at least progressive) change. However, recent critiques of human rights have stressed the neoliberal and moralizing aspects of such a universal framework (Brown 2004; Butler 2000; Žižek 2005). When applied to reproductive health in the global South, a human rights framework emphasizes the notion of choice. The poster of reproductive rights in the Introduction serves as an example. Women, once they are constructed as neoliberal individuals, become responsible for their health, their choice of contraception, and their choice of family size. Such a formulation of choice is at odds with the types of subjectivity and strategies I observed women and their networks of family enacting. Moreover, it erases the structural forces that significantly limit women's agency and ability to choose. To extend neoliberal responsibilities and their moral overtone to all of the women in my study would add insult to injury, for they were already subject to a global discourse about small, happy families that conflicted with local discourses about sons (and a patrilocal residence system). To expect women to be independent actors with a moral responsibility to make so-called good choices about their reproductive health is egregious, and to pretend they have the ability to truly choose their reproductive actions as if they were selecting which sari to wear that day is farcical.

The notions of freedom and choice are cultural constructs, celebrated myths, in much of the Western world. If, according to social theory, all choices are culturally influenced and structurally constrained, it does not make sense to strive for more choice. Likewise, if absolute social freedom means a lack of a social network for cooperation and support, why would one strive to have no obligations? The problem arises when familial relationships become so unequal or hierarchical that certain family members are able to exploit others with little or no consequence.

To conclude, I do not intend to pathologize patrilocality, for freedom from familial obligation is not the end goal—everyone has responsibilities to kin, and freeing oneself from those responsibilities would be as damaging as liberatory. Nonetheless, in this context it becomes clear that men have the upper hand and benefit more in this iteration of the patrilocal marriage system. Women are not disempowered because they suffer for others, prioritize others, or act dutifully towards their husbands or in-laws, yet their devotion takes these forms because structurally they are in a position of less power. While I am critical of the way a Western discourse of progress insidiously underlies much Western thinking, as Saba Mahmood incisively argues at length (2005), when I witness women suffering in their families, like Radha, or a young man suffering due to his economic status, like Dhan, and I know that suffering could be mitigated by a redistribution of power through social reform, I refuse to take a position of cultural relativism. Nepali scholars, artists, and activists witness and attempt to address these same issues. As an outsider, it is simply my hope to add to the conversation.

Conclusion: The Intimacies of Social Reproduction and Change

Based on ethnographic research from Hindu-caste Nepali families in a semi-urban village in the Kathmandu Valley, I describe the ways contemporary married women negotiated the globalized morality of the two-child family, the societal importance of sons, and their intimate familial relationships. Many cultural norms and modes of production that historically supported son preference were being questioned or left behind by contemporary couples, but a few remained salient: particularly the ideal of a multi-generational extended family. Mothers had new hopes for the future achievements of their daughters, but concomitantly they recognized that their daughters would be lost to other families though marriage and thus play a negligible role in the mother's future. Given this constraint, women worked to maintain a desirable set and form of supportive relationships—with husbands, sons, and daughters-in-law—through their projects of reproduction.

Despite changes in gender norms, education, and economic factors, young mothers ultimately subscribed to the patrilocal multi-generational joint family ideal, and reluctantly, to needing a son. And it turned out that sons—at least middle-class sons—still relied on the patrilocal extended family ideal as well. In an economy that cannot support sufficient job opportunities, educated young men felt that their society was letting them down. This, along with their experience of globality, seemed to heighten their awareness of the benefits offered by living with one's parents after marriage, seeing the joint family as a refuge from the struggles faced by men like Dhan or those who left Vishnupura to work abroad. If for married women the joint family system functioned to uphold the pressure to produce a son, for young men it offered a way to hold up their end of the patriarchal bargain. In order to support their future wives and children, they needed the assistance and support of their parents. Thus sons intended to remain living with their parents. I suspect their mothers will be happy to hear this conclusion.

APPENDIX A
CASTE HIERARCHY IN NEPAL

Wearers of the Sacred Thread
(*taagaadhari*)

Upadhyay Brahman
Rajput (Thakuri)
Jaisi Brahman
Chhetri
Newar Brahman
Indian Brahman
Ascetic sects
Various Newar castes

Non-enslaveable Alcohol Drinkers
(*namasinyaa matwaali*)

Magar
Gurung
Sunuwar
Some other Newar castes

Enslaveable Alcohol Drinkers
(*masinyaa matwaali*)

Bhote (people of Tibetan origin)
Chepang
Kumal (potters)
Tharu
Gharti (descendants of freed slaves)

Impure but Touchable
(*paani nachalnyaa choi chito haalnu naparnyaa*)

Kasai (Newar butchers)
Kusle (Newar musicians)
Hindu Dhobi (Newar washermen)
Musulman
Mlecch (Europeans)

Untouchable
(*paani nachalnyaa choi chito haalnu parcha*)

Kami (blacksmiths) and Sarki (tanners)
Damai (tailors and musicians)
Gaine (minstrels)
Badi (musicians and prostitutes)
Cyame (Newar scavengers)

Source: Adapted from *The Caste Hierarchy and the State in Nepal* (Hofer 1979).

APPENDIX B
TRENDS IN CONTRACEPTIVE
USE IN NEPAL

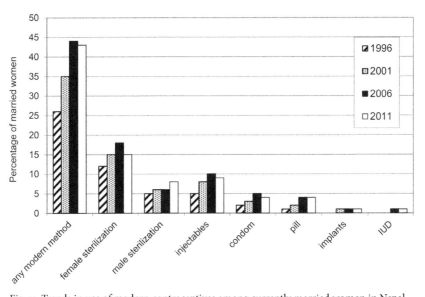

Fig. 11. Trends in use of modern contraceptives among currently married women in Nepal. *Source*: Adapted from Nepal Demographic and Health Survey 2011 (Ministry of Health and Population et al. 2012)

NOTES

Introduction

1 Liechty (2003) noted, however, that there was a considerable black market for international music in Kathmandu, with some young, urban men even keeping track of the top songs on the *Rolling Stone* charts. And several local boys in Vishnupura ran one-room rental shops of CDs and DVDs throughout the years of my research.

2 Although conspiracy theories abounded, the crowned Prince Dipendra was blamed for the shooting spree in the palace that killed much of the royal family. The prince then shot himself, and died shortly after being named King while in a coma. According to the rules of succession, Birendra's brother, Gyanendra, was thus next in line for the crown.

3 In April of 2007, the excombatants of the People's Liberation Army rejoined the government, moving back into mainstream politics. In September the Maoists (Communist Party of Nepal) left the interim government in order to apply pressure for the abolishment of the monarchy, and two months later rejoined as a result of Parliament approving the elimination of the monarchy.

4 For an analysis of student movements in Nepal during these years, see Snellinger (2007).

5 This was not the case, as stated previously, for people of high profile or people living in rural areas where the fighting was taking place, and one should not make generalizations about the levels of violence across Nepal based on my somewhat quiet, sheltered research area.

6 See Shneiderman (2004) and Turin and Pettigrew (2004) for firsthand accounts of rural areas during this period of time.

7 Intersectionality is the study of intersections amongst various social categories—such as gender, race, class, caste, or sexual orientation—and how such categories interact to create an individual's experience of social inequities. The sociological theory was coined by Kimberle Crenshaw (1989).

8 In doing so I do not intend to dismiss these debates, for they have added much theoretical richness to our understanding of how women negotiate power structures in various social contexts. Most influential to my thinking and arguments are a series of revelatory works on gender and agency: Abu-Lughod's *Veiled Sentiments*, Raheja

and Gold's *Listen to the Heron's Words*, Ellen Gruenbaum's article "Resistance and Embrace," Laura Ahearn's scholarship on agency, Holly Wardlow's *Wayward Women*, and Sherry Ortner's *Anthropology and Social Theory*. Without such a significant lineage of ideas about women's sources and expressions of power, I would not be in a position to attempt to further the discussion.

1   Intersections

1 In an effort to respect people's privacy, I use a pseudonym for the name of the community where this research is based. In previous publications I used the pseudonym Vishnumati, the name of a well-known river that runs through Kathmandu. I discovered that that name was too distracting to Nepali speakers, so I have switched it to Vishnupura.

2 In the initial planning stages of this research, I used census data from *Population of Nepal: Village Development Committees/Municipalities Population Census 2001*, published by the Central Bureau of Statistics in Kathmandu, to select a fieldwork site.

3 According to the Nepal census of 2001 (Central Bureau of Statistics 2002), the Hindu-caste community comprised almost 44 percent of the total population in Vishnupura.

4 There were two refusals. I excluded households in which one or more spouses were not Nepalese citizens.

5 Although many Newars are also Hindu and have castes, I excluded them from the case studies because they are culturally and linguistically distinct from the Parbatiya Hindu castes.

6 Meena Manandhar was instrumental to this research in many ways. First, as a woman it would have been culturally inappropriate in this location for me to walk around and call upon families alone. With another woman present, this behavior was fine. More importantly, Meena was a skilled interviewer with a Masters Degree in Anthropology. And, though I am conversationally fluent in Nepali, as a native speaker Meena had linguistic tact and grace that I lacked as an outsider. I was an active participant in the interview sessions, but she posed many of my questions for this reason. I crafted the interview schedule and translated the questions into Nepali and tested them with the help of another research assistant and native Nepali speaker, Manoj K. Shrestha. Throughout the book I use "we" instead of "I" in a few appropriate places because "I" would imply I was conducting interviews alone, whereas, in fact, it was a team effort. Meena and Manoj were not translators, in fact we conversed only in Nepali; rather they were key players in successfully carrying out my research.

7 The English word "caste" is an inadequate translation of the Nepali word *jaat*, but due to the lack of a better single-word translation, "caste" is used in this book for the sake of simplicity.

8 Household numbers (HH #) from my enumeration of households in 2003 are included to aid in keeping track of case studies and members of the same household.

9 In another context, India, Dirks has argued that Brahmins should not be considered at the top of the social hierarchy given that kings were not inferior to Brahmins. He argued that the political domain was not encompassed by a religious domain, and that purity and pollution were not the only significant factors of the Hindu caste hierarchy. He was responding to Dumont's treatise on caste, *Homo hierarchicus,* and the subsequent debate by scholars of India over ritual versus political status.

10 Since this family is one of very few low-caste, wealthy families in the community, a few inaccurate details are included to protect their identity. Those details are insignificant and plausible; they neither embellish nor subtract from the truth.

11 In part, I am responding here to Pradhan's article on measuring empowerment and women's reproductive health (2003). While I hold a different perspective on the definition of agency than Pradhan, following more closely that which was outlined by Bourdieu and Ahearn, I agree with and expand upon her rationale for needing in-depth anthropological research to address issues concerning women, power, and reproductive health.

2   Like a Potter's Wheel

1 See Kathryn March's book *"If Each Comes Halfway": Meeting Tamang Women in Nepal* (2002) for a model of allowing women to tell their own stories and the relevance of those stories to understanding social processes.

2 An increase in inter-caste and inter-ethnic group marriages is altering the experience of marriage captured by these women's stories.

3 A further explanation of *ghar* follows in the text.

4 The label "homebirth" should be recognized as a recent Western construct developed in opposition to the relatively recent dominant category of "hospital birth." The term homebirth does not capture adequately the ways birth occurred historically in Nepal, for sometimes births happened in agricultural fields, on the path, in a cowshed, in a garden, etcetera.

5 See also Bennett (1982); Croll (2000); Das Gupta (1995); Jeffery, Jeffery and Lyon (1988). For differences between low- and high-caste Nepali families see Cameron (1998).

6 In order to ensure that the family remains unidentifiable I will not provide details to explain, but a history of two previous wives (no longer present) and their children (who were present) complicated the kinship relations within this household.

7 *JeTho, mailo, sailo, kaanchho* (and there are more if needed) are all adjectives that designate the birth order of children. In the case of buhaaris in a joint family, it is the birth order of the son to whom the buhaari is married that determines whether they are *jeThi* buhaari, etcetera.

8 A system of labor exchange in which a person works in another person's fields, but sometimes for grain or cash rather than exchange of labor.

9 For a study of gender and mobility in the Kathmandu Valley amongst young, unmarried women see my article, "'Scooty Girls': Mobility and Intimacy at the Margins of Kathmandu" (2014).

3 The Elusive Small, Happy Family

1 In line with Judith Justice's critique of bureaucratic institutions in *Policies, Plans, and People*, I do not intend to criticize the intentions or motivations of individual people, but rather draw attention to the collective goals as stated in program outlines.

2 For a critique specifically addressing demography in this regard, see Riley (1999).

3 Errington (1990) summarizes how feminist agendas moved from universal questions, categories, and arguments toward considering particular contexts. Women of different classes, ethnicities, and sexual preferences protested the homogenizing and universalizing category of "women" as it had been constructed by Euro-American feminists. As di Leonardo wrote, feminist scholars were forced to confront ". . . the question of 'difference'—the multiple racial, ethnic, class, sexual, age, regional, and national identities of women—as they noted their own restricted demographic representation and research interests" (1991, 18). Prior to that point, women had been discussed as if they were a unified assemblage—as if being female alone was uniting enough to bind them together in a definitive group.

4 This time period is used, rather than newer statistics, because it is roughly the time when women in this study were giving birth.

4 Son Preference and the Preferences of Sons

1 If their class status was noticeably privileged or disadvantaged, I mention it in the following text. In cases where the young men's class status was less marked and somewhere in the middle, I refrain from mentioning it. My estimation of class was based on whether their family owns or rents a home, ownership of a television, computer, motorbike, or car, along with symbols such as dress, speech, and mobile phones (which can be manipulated by individuals, but only to an extent), their employment, and their level of education. All of these are locally appropriate markers of class. And as I discussed previously, "class" mostly captures markers of disposable income and is not a reliable category in this context. Families with significant wealth tied up in land holdings may have very little disposable income to spend on clothes and mobile phones, while a family who recently sold their land might have a large influx of cash that is depleted relatively quickly on consumer items rather than saved for the long term.

2 Note that the numbers inserted after the first person who speaks in each quote refer to the number assigned to the group interview. For example, Dev was a member of the second group I interviewed. I have included the numbers to assist in keeping track of which young men are speaking and of which group they were a part.

3 The literal translation of the proverb is, "Whichever yogi comes, (he has) pierced ears."

4 See also Craig Jeffrey's (2010) extended treatment of this topic in India in his book *Timepass: Youth, Class, and the Politics of Waiting in India*.

5   Conclusion

1 Rahman's (1999) longitudinal study in Bangladesh discusses how having two
  sons significantly improved parental survival due to the fact that having two
  sons increased options for parents when one of them was unreliable or had a low
  income.

REFERENCES

Abu-Lughod, Lila. 1986. *Veiled Sentiments*. Berkeley: University of California Press.
———. 1993. *Writing Women's Worlds: Bedouin Stories*. Berkeley: University of California Press.
Ahearn, Laura. 2001a. *Invitations to Love: Literacy, Love Letters, and Social Change in Nepal*. Ann Arbor: University of Michigan Press.
———. 2001b. "Language and Agency." *Annual Review of Anthropology* 30: 109–137.
Appadurai, Arjun, ed. 1988. *The Social Life of Things: Commodities in Cultural Perspective*. Cambridge: Cambridge University Press.
———. 1991. "Global Ethnoscapes: Notes and Queries for a Transnational Anthropology." In *Recapturing Anthropology*, edited by Richard Fox, 191–210. Santa Fe: School of American Research Press.
Axinn, William G. 1992. "Family Organization and Fertility Limitation in Nepal." *Demography* 29 (4): 503–521.
Axinn, William G. and Scott T. Yabiku. 2001. "Social Change, the Social Organization of Families, and Fertility Limitation." *American Journal of Sociology* 106 (5): 1219–1261.
Barker, Carol E., Cherry E. Bird, Ajit Pradhan, and Ganga Shakya. 2007. "Support to the Safe Motherhood Programme in Nepal: An Integrated Approach." *Reproductive Health Matters* 15 (30): 81–90.
Bayly, Susan. 1999. *Caste, Society, and Politics in India from the Eighteenth Century to the Modern Age*. Cambridge: Cambridge University Press.
Bennett, Lynn. 1982. *Dangerous Wives and Sacred Sisters: Social and Symbolic Roles of High-Caste Women in Nepal*. New York: Columbia University Press.
Besnier, Niko. 2011. *On the Edge of the Global: Modern Anxieties in a Pacific Island Nation*. Stanford: Stanford University Press.
Biehl, Joao. 2007. *Will to Live: AIDS Therapies and the Politics of Survival*. Princeton: Princeton University Press.
Bledsoe, Caroline. 2002. *Contingent Lives: Fertility, Time, and Aging in West Africa*. Chicago: University of Chicago Press.
Bossen, Laurel. 2007. "Village to Distant Village: The Opportunities and Risks of Long-distance Marriage Migration in Rural China." *Journal of Contemporary China* 16 (50): 97–116.

Bourdieu, Pierre. 1977. *Outline of a Theory of Practice*. Cambridge: Cambridge University Press.

Bradley, Candice. 1995. "Women's Empowerment and Fertility Decline in Western Kenya." In *Situating Fertility: Anthropology and Demographic Inquiry*, edited by Susan Greenhalgh, 157–178. Cambridge: Cambridge University Press.

Brown, Wendy. 2004. " "The Most We Can Hope for . . .": Human Rights and the Politics of Fatalism." *The South Atlantic Quarterly* 103 (2/3): 451–463.

Browner, Carole, and Carolyn Sargent. 2011. "Introduction: Toward Global Anthropological Studies of Reproduction: Concepts, Methods, Theoretical Approaches." In *Reproduction, Globalization, and the State*, edited by Carole Browner and Carolyn Sargent, 1–17. Durham: Duke University Press.

Brunson, Jan. 2010a. "Son Preference in the Context of Fertility Decline: Limits to New Constructions of Gender and Kinship in Nepal." *Studies in Family Planning* 41 (2): 89–98.

———. 2010b. "Confronting Maternal Mortality, Controlling Birth in Nepal: The Gendered Politics of Receiving Biomedical Care at Birth." *Social Science and Medicine* 71 (10): 1719–1727.

———. 2011. "Moving Away from Marital Violence: Nepali Mothers Who Refuse to Stay." *Practicing Anthropology* 33 (3): 17–21.

———. 2013. "A Review of Women's Health: The Hegemony of Caste, Development, and Biomedicine." *Studies in Nepali History and Society* 18 (2): 279–303.

———. 2014. " 'Scooty Girls': Mobility and Intimacy at the Margins of Kathmandu." *Ethnos* 79 (5): 610–629.

Brunson, Jan, and Zakea Boeger. n.d. "Guerilla, Mother, Wife: The Personal Politics of Fighting for Gender Equity in Maoist Revolutions." Unpublished manuscript.

Butler, Judith. 2000. "Restaging the Universal: Hegemony and the Limits of Formalism." In *Contingency, Hegemony, Universality: Contemporary Dialogues on the Left*, edited by Judith Butler, Ernesto Laclau and Slavoj Zizek, 11–43. New York: Verso.

Caldwell, John C. 1982. "The Wealth Flows Theory of Fertility Decline." In *Theory of Fertility Decline*, edited by John Caldwell, 333–351. New York: Academic Press.

———. 1998. "The Global Fertility Transition and Nepal." *Contributions to Nepalese Studies* 25: 1–7.

Cameron, Mary M. 1998. *On the Edge of the Auspicious: Gender and Caste in Nepal*. Chicago: University of Illinois Press.

Carter, Anthony T. 1995. "Agency and Fertility: For an Ethnography of Practice." In *Situating Fertility: Anthropology and Demographic Inquiry*, edited by Susan Greenhalgh, 55–85. Cambridge: Cambridge University Press.

Central Bureau of Statistics. 2002. Population of Nepal: Village Development Committees/Municipalities Population Census 2001. Kathmandu.

Chatterjee, Nilanjana and Nancy E. Riley. 2001. "Planning an Indian Modernity: The Gendered Politics of Fertility Control." *Signs* 26 (3): 811–845.

Comaroff, Jean and John Comaroff. 2011. *Theory from the South: Or, How Euro-America is Evolving Toward Africa*. Boulder: Paradigm Publishers.

Connelly, Matthew. 2003. "Population Control is History: New Perspectives on the International Campaign to Limit Population Growth." *Comparative Studies in Society and History* 45 (01): 122–147.

Crenshaw, Kimberle. 1989. "Demarginalizing the Intersection of Race and Sex." *University of Chicago Legal Forum* 139–167.

———. 1991. "Mapping the Margins: Intersectionality, Identity Politics, and Violence Against Women of Color." *Stanford Law Review* 43 (1241): 1241–1299.

Croll, Elisabeth. 2000. *Endangered Daughters: Discrimination and Development in Asia.* New York: Routledge.

Csordas, Thomas J. 1990. "Embodiment as a Paradigm for Anthropology." *Ethos* 18 (1): 5–47.

———. 1999. "The Body's Career in Anthropology." In *Anthropological Theory Today*, edited by Henrietta L. Moore, 172–205. Boston: Polity.

Das, Veena. 1992. "Reflections on the Social Construction of Adulthood." In *Identity and Adulthood*, edited by Sudhir Kakar, 89–104. Delhi: Oxford University Press.

Das Gupta, Monica. 1995. "Lifecourse Perspectives on Women's Autonomy and Health Outcomes." *American Anthropologist* 97 (3): 481–491.

———. 1997. "Kinship Systems and Demographic Regimes." In Anthropological Demography, edited by David I. Kertzer and Tom Fricke, 36–52. Chicago: University of Chicago Press.

de Sousa Santos, Boaventura. 2008. "Introduction: Opening Up the Canon of Knowledge and Recognition of Difference." In *Another Knowledge is Possible: Beyond Northern Epistemologies*, edited by Boaventura de Sousa Santos, xix–lxii. Brooklyn: Verso.

di Leonardo, Micaela. 1991. "Introduction: Gender, Culture, and Political Economy: Feminist Anthropology in Historical Perspective." In *Gender at the Crossroads of Knowledge*, edited by Micaela di Leonardo, 1–48. Berkeley: University of California Press.

Dyson, Tim and Mick Moore. 1983. "On Kinship Structure, Female Autonomy, and Demographic Behavior in India." *Population and Development Review* 9 (1): 35–60.

Ehrlich, Paul. 1968. *The Population Bomb.* New York: Ballantine Books.

Errington, Shelly. 1990. "Recasting Sex, Gender, and Power: A Theoretical and Regional Overview." In *Power and Difference: Gender in Island Southeast Asia*, edited by Jane Monnig Atkinson and Shelly Errington, 1–58. Stanford: Stanford University Press.

Escobar, Arturo. 1995. *Encountering Development: The Making and Unmaking of the Third World.* Princeton: Princeton University Press.

Farmer, Paul. 1999. *Infections and Inequalities: The Modern Plagues.* Berkeley: University of California Press.

Ferguson, James. 1997. "Anthropology and Its Evil Twin 'Development' in the Constitution of a Discipline." In *International Development and the Social Sciences*, edited by Frederick Cooper and Randall M. Packard, 150–175. Berkeley: University of California Press.

Fordyce, Lauren. 2012. "Responsible Choices: Situating Pregnancy Intention among Haitians in South Florida." *Medical Anthropology Quarterly* 26 (1): 116–135.

Foucault, Michel. 1978. *The History of Sexuality: An Introduction.* New York: Random House.

Fricke, Tom. 1994. *Himalayan Households: Tamang Demography and Domestic Processes.* New York: Columbia University Press.

Fruzzetti, Lina. 1982. *The Gift of the Virgin.* New Brunswick: Rutgers University Press.

Fruzzetti, Lina, Akos Ostor, and Steve Barnett. 1992. "The Cultural Construction of the Person in Bengal and Tamilnadu." In *Concepts of Person: Kinship, Caste, and Marriage in India,* edited by Lina Fruzzetti, Akos Ostor and Steve Barnett, 8–30. Delhi: Oxford University Press.

Fujikura, Tatsuro. 2004. "Vasectomies and Other Engagements with Modernity: A Reflection on Discourses and Practices of Family Planning in Nepal." *Journal of the Japanese Association for South Asian Studies* 16: 40–71.

Ginsburg, Faye D. and Rayna Rapp. 1995. "Introduction: Conceiving the New World Order." In *Conceiving the New World Order: The Global Politics of Reproduction,* edited by Faye D. Ginsburg and Rayna Rapp, 1–19. Berkeley: University of California Press.

Government of Nepal. 1992. *Eighth Plan (1992–1997).* Kathmandu: National Planning Commission.

———. 1997. *Ninth Plan (1997–2002).* Kathmandu: National Planning Commission.

Greenhalgh, Susan. 1990. "Toward a Political Economy of Fertility: Anthropological Contributions." *Population and Development Review* 16 (1): 85–106.

———. 1994. "Controlling Births and Bodies in Village China." American Ethnologist 21 (1): 3–30.

———. 1995. "Anthropology Theorizes Reproduction: Integrating Practice, Political Economy, and Feminist Perspectives." In *Situating Fertility: Anthropology and Demographic Inquiry,* edited by Susan Greenhalgh, 3–28. Cambridge: Cambridge University Press.

———. 1996. "The Social Construction of Population Science: An Intellectual, Institutional, and Political History of Twentieth-Century Demography." *Comparative Studies in Society and History* 38 (1): 26–66.

Gruenbaum, Ellen. 1998. "Resistance and Embrace: Sudanese Rural Women and Systems of Power." In *Pragmatic Women and Body Politics,* edited by Margaret Lock and Patricia Kaufert, 58–76. Cambridge: Cambridge University Press.

Guneratne, Arjun. 2001. "Shaping the Tourist's Gaze: Representing Ethnic Difference in a Nepali Village." *Journal of the Royal Anthropological Institute* 7 (3): 527–543.

———. 2002. Many Tongues, One People: The Making of Tharu Identity in Nepal. Ithaca: Cornell University Press.

Hangen, Susan. 2005. "Race and the Politics of Identity in Nepal." *Ethnology* 44 (1): 49–64.

———. 2010. *The Rise of Ethnic Politics in Nepal.* New York: Routledge.

Hartmann, Betsy. 1995. *Reproductive Rights and Wrongs: The Global Politics of Population Control.* Boston: South End Press.

Hofer, Andras. 1979. *The Caste Hierarchy and the State in Nepal: A Study of the Muluki Ain of 1854.* Innsbruck: Universitatsverlag Wagner.

Jeffery, Craig. 2010. *Timepass: Youth, Class, and the Politics of Waiting in India.* Stanford: Stanford University Press.

Jeffery, Patricia, Roger Jeffery, and Andrew Lyon. 1988. *Labour Pains and Labour Power.* London and New Delhi: Zed Books Ltd.

Jeffery, Roger and Patricia Jeffery. 1997. *Population, Gender, and Politics: Demographic Change in Rural North India.* Cambridge: Cambridge University Press.

Justice, Judith. 1989. *Policies, Plans, and People.* Berkeley: University of California Press.

Kertzer, David I. and Thomas E. Fricke. 1997. "Towards an Anthropological Demography." In *Anthropological Demography: Toward a New Synthesis,* edited by David I. Kertzer and Thomas E. Fricke, 1–35. Chicago: Chicago University Press.

Kunreuther, Laura. 2006. "Technologies of the Voice: FM Radio, Telephone, and the Nepali Diaspora in Kathmandu." *Cultural Anthropology* 21 (3): 323–353.

Lamb, Sarah. 2000. *White Saris and Sweet Mangoes: Aging, Gender, and Body in North India.* Berkeley: University of California Press.

Lawoti, Mahendra, and Susan Hangen, eds. 2013. *Nationalism and Ethnic Conflict in Nepal: Identities and Mobilization after 1990.* New York: Routledge.

Liechty, Mark. 2003. *Suitably Modern: Making Middle-Class Culture in a New Consumer Society.* Princeton: Princeton University Press.

Mahmood, Saba. 2005. *Politics of Piety: The Islamic Revival and the Feminist Subject.* Princeton: Princeton University Press.

March, Kathryn. 2002. *"If Each Comes Halfway": Meeting Tamang Women in Nepal.* Ithaca: Cornell University.

Marcus, George and Michael Fischer. 1986. *Anthropology as Cultural Critique: An Experimental Moment in the Human Sciences.* Chicago: University of Chicago Press.

Mason, Karen Oppenheim. 1986. "The Status of Women: Conceptual and Methodological Issues in Demographic Studies." *Sociological Forum* 1 (2): 284–299.

———. 1987. "The Impact of Women's Social Position on Fertility in Developing Countries." *Sociological Forum* 2 (4): 718–745.

———. 1995. "Review of 'Reproductive Rights and Wrongs: The Global Politics of Population Control (Revised Edition)' by Betsy Hartmann." *Population & Development Review* 21 (4): 885–887.

Maternowska, M. Catherine. 2006. *Reproducing Inequities: Poverty and the Politics of Population in Haiti.* New Brunswick: Rutgers University Press.

McNicoll, Geoffrey. 1995. "On Population Growth and Revisionism: Further Questions." *Population & Development Review* 21 (2): 307–340.

Mines, Diane. 2009. *Caste in India.* Ann Arbor: Association for Asian Studies.

Ministry of Health and Population, New ERA, and ICF International Inc. 2012. Nepal Demographic and Health Survey 2011. Kathmandu.

Ministry of Health and Population, New ERA, and Macro International Inc. 2007. Nepal Demographic and Health Survey 2006. Kathmandu.

Ministry of Health and Population, New ERA, and ORC Macro. 2002. Nepal Demographic and Health Survey 2001. Calverton, Maryland.

Mishra, Chaitanya and Om Gurung, eds. 2012. *Ethnicity and Federalisation in Nepal.* Kathmandu: Department of Sociology/Anthropology, Tribhuvan University.

Mohanty, Chandra Talpade. 1984. "Under Western Eyes: Feminist Scholarship and Colonial Discourses." *boundary 2* 12 (3): 333–358.

———. 2003. ""Under Western Eyes" Revisited: Feminist Solidarity through Anticapitalist Struggles." *Signs* 28 (2): 499–535.

Mol, Anne Marie. 2003. *The Body Multiple: Ontology in Medical Practice.* Durham: Duke University Press.

Mullany, Britta C. 2006. "Barriers to and Attitudes towards Promoting Husbands' Involvement in Maternal Health in Katmandu, Nepal." *Social Science & Medicine* 62 (11): 2798–2809.

Mullany, Britta C., B. Lakhey, D. Shrestha, Michelle J. Hindin, and Stan Becker. 2009. "Impact of Husbands' Participation in Antenatal Health Education on Maternal Health Knowledge." *Journal of Nepal Medical Association* 48 (173): 28–34.

Nightingale, Andrea J. 2011. "Bounding Difference: Intersectionality and the Material Production of Gender, Caste, Class and Environment in Nepal." *Geoforum* 42 (2): 153–162.

Niraula, Bhanu B. and S. Philip Morgan. 1996. "Marriage Formation, Post-Marital Contact with Natal Kin and Autonomy of Women: Evidence from Two Nepali Settings." *Population Studies* 50 (1): 35–50.

Ortner, Sherry. 1984. "Theory in Anthropology Since the Sixties." *Comparative Studies in Society and History* 26 (1): 126–166.

———. 1995. "Resistance and the Problem of Ethnographic Refusal." *Comparative Studies in Society and History* 37 (1): 173–193.

———. 2006. *Anthropology and Social Theory: Culture, Power, and the Acting Subject.* Durham: Duke University Press.

Paxson, Heather. 2002. "Rationalizing Sex: Family Planning and the Making of Modern Lovers in Urban Greece." *American Ethnologist* 29 (2): 307–334.

Petryna, Adryana, Andrew Lakoff, and Arthur Kleinman, eds. 2006. *Global Pharmaceuticals: Ethics, Markets, Practices.* Durham: Duke University Press.

Pettigrew, Judith. 2004. "Living Between the Maoists and the Army in Rural Nepal." In *Himalayan People's War*, edited by Michael Hutt, 261–283. Bloomington: Indiana University Press.

Pigg, Stacy Leigh. 1992. "Inventing Social Categories through Place: Social Representations and Development in Nepal." *Comparative Studies in Society and History* 34 (3): 491–513.

———. 1996. "The Credible and the Credulous: The Question of 'Villagers' Beliefs' in Nepal." *Cultural Anthropology* 11 (2): 160–201.

Pigg, Stacy Leigh and Vincanne Adams. 2005. "Introduction: The Moral Object of Sex." In *Sex in Development: Science, Sexuality, and Morality in Global Perspective*, 1–18. Durham: Duke University Press.

Pradhan, Bina. 2003. "Measuring Empowerment: A Methodological Approach." *Development* 46 (2): 51–57.

———. 2006. "Gender and Human Development." In *Nepal: Readings in Human Development*, edited by Sriram Raj Pande, Shawna Tropp, Bikash Sharma, and Yuba Raj Khatiwada, 81–115. Kathmandu: United Nations Development Programme.

Raheja, Gloria Goodwin and Ann Grodzins Gold. 1994. *Listen to the Heron's Words: Reimagining Gender and Kinship in North India.* Berkeley: University of California Press.

Rahman, Omar. 1999. "Family Matters: The Impact of Kin on the Mortality of the Elderly in Rural Bangladesh." *Population Studies* 53 (2): 227–235.

Riley, Nancy E. 1999. "Challenging Demography: Contributions from Feminist Theory." *Sociological Forum* 14 (3): 369–397.

Robertson, Roland. 1995. "Glocalization: Time-Space Homogeneity-Heterogeneity." In *Global Modernities*, edited by Mike Featherstone, Scott Lash, and Roland Robertson, 25–44. Thousand Oaks: Sage Publications Inc.

Robertson, Thomas. 2012. *The Malthusian Moment: Global Population Growth and the Birth of American Environmentalism.* New Brunswick: Rutgers University Press.

Romney, A. Kimball, Susan C. Weller, and William H. Batchelder. 1986. "Culture as Consensus: A Theory of Culture and Informant Accuracy." *American Anthropologist* 88 (2): 313–338.

Scheper-Hughes, Nancy and Margaret Lock. 1987. "The Mindful Body: A Prolegomenon to Future Work in Medical Anthropology." *Medical Anthropology Quarterly* 1 (1): 6–41.

Scott, James. 1999. *Seeing Like a State: How Certain Schemes to Improve the Human Condition Have Failed.* New Haven: Yale University Press.

Sen, Amartya. 1990. "More Than 100 Million Women Are Missing." *New York Review of Books* 20: 61–66.

Sharpless, John. 1997. "Population Science, Private Foundations, and Development Aid." In *International Development and the Social Sciences: Essays on the History and Politics of Knowledge*, edited by Frederick Cooper and Randall M. Packard, 176–202. Berkeley: University of California Press.

Shneiderman, Sara and Mark Turin. 2004. "The Path to *Jan Sarkar* in Dolakha District." In *Himalayan People's War*, edited by Michael Hutt, 79–111. Bloomington: Indiana University Press.

Skerry, Christa, Kerry Moran, and Kay Calavan. 1992 [1991]. Four Decades of Development: The History of U.S. Assistance to Nepal. Kathmandu: USAID/Nepal.

Skinner, William G. 1997. "Family Systems and Demographic Processes." In *Anthropological Demography*, edited by David I. Kertzer and Tom Fricke, 53–95. Chicago: University of Chicago Press.

Smith, Andrea. 2005. *Conquest: Sexual Violence and American Indian Genocide.* Brooklyn: South End Press.

Smith, Daniel Jordan. 2005. "Cell Phones, Sharing, and Social Status in an African Society." In *Applying Anthropology*, edited by Aaron Podolefsky and Peter J. Brown, 305–312. New York: McGraw-Hill.

Snellinger, Amanda. 2007. "Student Movements in Nepal: Their Parameters and their Idealized Forms." In *Contentious Politics and Democratization in Nepal*, edited by Mahendra Lawoti, 273–295. Delhi: Sage Publications.

Steger, Manfred. 2008. *The Rise of the Global Imaginary: Political Ideologies from the French Revolution to the Global War on Terror.* New York: Oxford University Press.

———. 2009. *Globalization: A Very Short Introduction.* 2nd ed. New York: Oxford University Press.

Stone, Pamela. 2008. *Opting Out? Why Women Really Quit Careers and Head Home.* Berkeley: University of California Press.

Tamang, Seira. 2002. "The Politics of "Developing Nepali Women."" In *The State of Nepal*, edited by Kanak Mani Dixit and Shastri Ramachandaran, 161–175. Kathmandu: Himal Books.

Tan, Lin and Susan E. Short. 2004. "Living as Double Outsiders: Migrant Women's Experiences of Marriage in a County-Level City." In *On the Move: Women and Rural-to-Urban Migration in Contemporary China*, edited by Arianne M. Gaetano and Tamara Jacka, 151–174. New York: Columbia University Press.

Thompson, Charis. 2007. *Making Parents: The Ontological Choreography of Reproductive Technologies*. Cambridge: MIT Press.

Thornton, Arland and Thomas E. Fricke. 1987. "Social Change and the Family: Comparative Perspectives from the West, China, and South Asia." *Sociological Forum* 2 (4): 746–749.

Trouillot, Michel-Rolph. 1995. *Silencing the Past: Power and the Production of History*. Boston: Beacon Press.

Tsing, Anna. 2000. "The Global Situation." *Cultural Anthropology* 15 (3): 327–360.

———. 2004. *Friction: An Ethnography of Global Connection*. Princeton: Princeton University Press.

United Nations Population Fund. 1994. "Advancing the Goals of the ICPD and the Millennium Summit." United Nations Population Fund, accessed March 15. http://www.unfpa.org/icpd.

Van Hollen, Cecilia. 2013. *Birth in the Age of AIDS*. Stanford: Stanford University Press.

Vatuk, Sylvia. 1975. "Gifts and Affines in North India." *Contributions to Indian Sociology* 9 (2): 155–196.

Vera-Sanso, Penny. 2004. " 'They Don't Need It, and I Can't Give It': Filial Support in South India." In *Ageing Without Children: European and Asian Perspectives on Elderly Access to Support Networks,* edited by Phillip Kreager and Schroder-Butterfill, 77–105. New York: Berghan Books.

Wardlow, Holly. 2006. *Wayward Women: Sexuality and Agency in a New Guinea Society.* Berkeley: University of California Press.

Weiss, Linda. 1999. "Single Women in Nepal: Familial Support, Familial Neglect." *Journal of Comparative Family Studies* 30 (2): 243–257.

World Bank, and DFID. 2006. Unequal Citizens: Gender, Caste, and Ethnic Exclusion in Nepal. Kathmandu.

Žižek, Slavoj. 2005. "Against Human Rights." New Left Review 34 (2): 115–131.

INDEX

Page numbers in *italics* represent figures.

ABOUT THE AUTHOR

JAN BRUNSON (Ph.D., Brown University, 2008) is an assistant professor in the Department of Anthropology at the University of Hawai'i at Manoa. She is an affiliate faculty member in the Department of Women's Studies and the Center for South Asian Studies. Her research intertwines medical anthropology, gender studies, and cultural studies of science, technology, and medicine. She has conducted ethnographic research in Nepal on women's health and the politics of reproduction for over a decade. Her research portfolio includes studies of contraceptive technologies and family planning discourses, maternal health in resource-poor settings, Maoist motherhood, and women's autonomy and spatial mobility. Her articles appear in the journals *Social Science and Medicine, Ethnos, Studies in Family Planning, Practicing Anthropology,* and *Studies in Nepali History and Society.*

CPSIA information can be obtained
at www.ICGtesting.com
Printed in the USA
LVOW01s1314271216
518836LV00023B/491/P